T0063428

GROWN MEN DON'T *Cry*

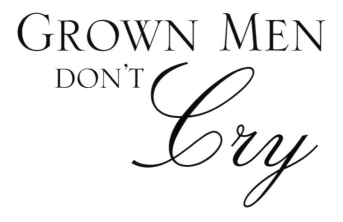

A Personal Journey of Despair and Hope

MICHAEL J. ROBERTS

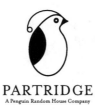

PARTRIDGE
A Penguin Random House Company

ISBN:	Hardcover	978-1-4828-9950-4
	Softcover	978-1-4828-9948-1
	eBook	978-1-4828-9949-8

To order additional copies of this book, contact
Toll Free 800 101 2657 (Singapore)
Toll Free 1 800 81 7340 (Malaysia)
orders.singapore@partridgepublishing.com

www.partridgepublishing.com/singapore

This book is dedicated to those
who are currently suffering from Cancer
~ there is hope and light at the end of the tunnel.

Join us in the cause and fight the good fight.
We can make that needed difference
in the lives of so many.

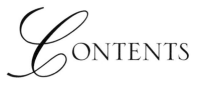

ONTENTS

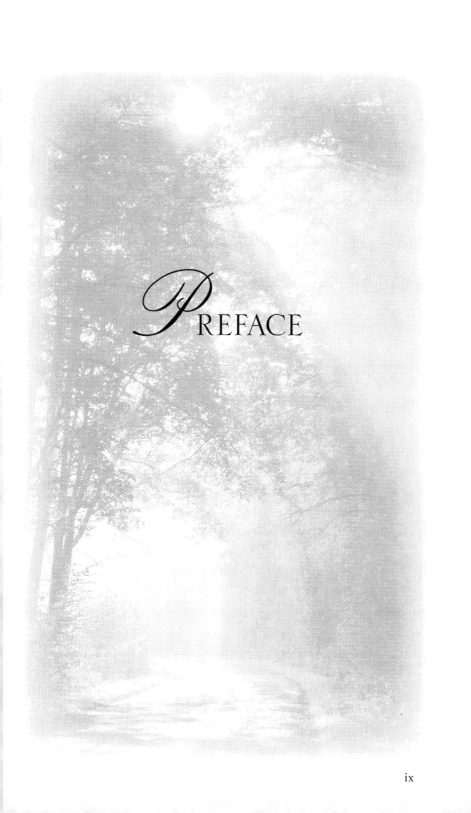

PREFACE

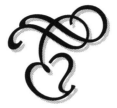

God has a Plan for each and every one of us. However we as humble beings often wonder what this plan is, and if the greater the suffering, one would think the greater the rewards.

I remember my mother telling me as a young boy in England: "Grow Up, Act like a Man."

I can recall how poor we were and from the age of 7 years I would be forced to work in the fields picking peas, potatoes and whatever instead of attending school just so we had money to live on. My stepfather was very hard on the children and wanted to make a man out of me. Nothing like that was ever said to my two elder sisters—June and Angela—it was a man's world and grown men don't cry.

Even when I left school at the age of 14, moved out of the family home and had my own lodging, I often wondered what was in store for me. What was my life's plan? At that time, we only went to Church on Sundays to collect food and hand-me-down clothes, so I never had much faith in the Church, let alone God.

I moved to greener pastures at the age of 20 and bought a one-way air ticket to Christchurch, New Zealand. I found myself in a strange country living with my grandparents whom I could never remember seeing before in my younger years, but there I was starting out not knowing what my plans were and what life would offer me.

Of course as a young 20-year-old, one tries out many of life's challenges: drinking, partying, dating, driving fast cars (well trying to get old cars to drive fast) until I got into trouble and was "redirected" into making a choice to join the Army and become a real man or end up in real trouble—hence I was soon given a haircut (shave) dressed in greens and was told "You become a Man and Grown Men Don't Cry". Now where did I hear that phrase before?

After completing 20 years of professional service in the New Zealand Army (retired from service as Senior Warrant Officer) and having served on tour in Singapore (1976-78, & 1991) I had learnt the art of wearing one's mask. If you had to "drill" something into a young recruit, much like a Senior Warrant officer having to drill something into a young officer, I would wear my "mask" and become a man of steel in order to teach a lesson and drive home the point. I would find myself preaching these words "Grown Men Don't Cry"—to make the cadet a 'hardened' soldier and encourage him to also wear a mask in order to hide his tears of pain.

The real lesson one learns is that *Grown Men Do Cry* and I only found that out at the age of 55 when I was told I had late Stage 3 Cancer, and needed a major operation in order to live.

One's life training and wearing one's mask came automatically and having just completed a catechism course to join the Catholic Church, I was in the mist of finding God and knowing what his plan might be for me. The familiar words of a hymn "In His Time" struck me poignantly . . .

In His time, in His time
He makes all things beautiful in His time
Lord, please show me everyday
As You're teaching me Your Way
And I'll do just what you say
In Your time.

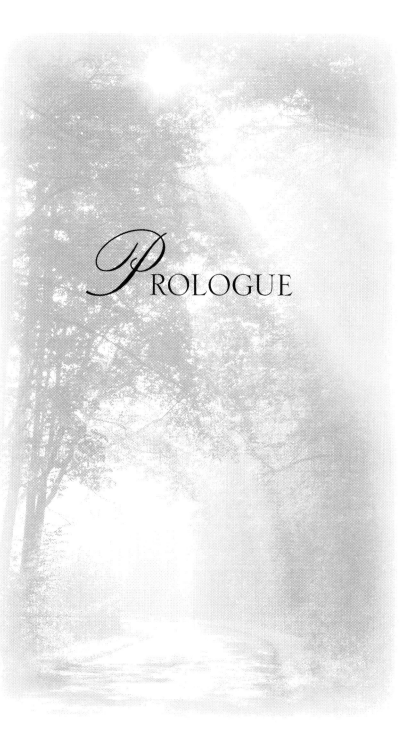

PROLOGUE

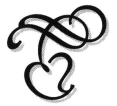

Father come to me, hold me up 'cause I can barely stand
My strength is gone and my breath is short, I can't
Reach out my hands
But my heart is set on a pilgrimage to heaven's own bright King
So in faltering or victory I will always sing

These are some of the words I was hearing while I lay in a hospital bed dressed in a white operating gown— all prepped for the main event of my life—outside the main Operating theatre of Tan Tock Seng Hospital (TTSH). The hospital was located 10 minutes from our home, picked only because it was located nearby and it was like our regular 'family' hospital, where I had been treated for eye problems and other health issues, not for the excellent record of treating cancer patients. To me, one doctor is as good as another, unless you have the money to "buy" the very best. One just has to accept how the cards fall.

It had not struck me that I was about to face the most challenging stage of my life, and how major the surgery would be. I was told an insertion here (stomach) and an insertion there (back area) and we have a look inside and see what we can find, so I expected that it would be over and done with within a few hours, and the following week I would be up and about and being the grumpy old man that I am.

I can recall my wife, Karen, being as optimistic as ever; my eldest son, Shaun (who had changed his name to Chris) age 30, had flown in from New Zealand and stood like a rock as I heard him say "The Roberts's are fighters, he be ok". I remember during the initial days, how my oldest daughter Sharon (age 25) was very upset and found it hard to talk, my youngest son Shane (age 21) was quiet and supportive, while my youngest daughter Michelle (age 7) was the most concerned holding my hand and trying to give me assurance—all their emotions were very real to me; I had my whole family with me and I was happy and at peace so even if I did not make it (30% chance of success) I was at least at peace.

I was admitted to the hospital on the 28 November 2010, went through all the pre-Op procedures, said my goodbyes and was wheeled to the Pre-Op room. I waited for almost an hour only to be told there was no ICU room available, hence no operation would take place. I needed to go back home and the operation would be re-scheduled for another day, now how's that for stress?!

As my situation was a very urgent case we managed to re-schedule the operation for 2 December 2010 after paying an extra S$3,000 for the ICU room on top of the S$8,000 deposit for the Operation. 2 Dec came quickly and hence the re-run of Pre-Op preparation and the goodbyes were undertaken a second time. It was routine for them to ask my name and Singapore identity card number an endless number of times, and also the endless queries if I had fasted. Well, I had not eaten for at least 8 hours and had been briefed about what was about to happen in the Operating room. At this point I had very little to say. My mind was racing and I tried to 'blank' out all things related to the operation. Without a doubt this was going to be a major surgery, the surgeons had briefed me that they would be removing part of my gullet and my stomach. It was not until later that I found out how major the operation was and that my gall bladder had also been removed (I remember one of the surgeons, saying this by my bedside after the operation, that they felt they might as well take out the gall bladder while they were inside). Who knows what else they removed while they were fishing inside of me . . .

I had to learn fast about Cancer and what it was all about; the different stages and sub—stages, how it spreads via the lymph nodes, on-going treatment like radiation and chemotherapy which one does not fully realise what it does to your body unless it is happening to you, and when/if it does, most of us would be numbed.

Here's a brief summary of what the four stages of Cancer means for most types of Cancer:

> **Stage One** usually means the cancer is relatively small and contained within the organ it started in.
>
> **Stage Two** usually means the cancer has not started to spread into surrounding tissues, but the

tumour is larger than in Stage One. Sometimes it means the cancer cells may have started to spread into the lymph nodes close to the tumour.

Stage Three usually means the cancer is larger. It may have started to spread into surrounding tissues and there are cancer cells in the lymph nodes in the area and away from the actual tumour.

Stage Four means the cancer has spread from where it started to another body organ and is commonly called the secondary cancer.

In each stage there are four sub-stages. In my case I was diagnosed with Stage Three, sub-Stage Four cancer of the Oesophagus (three tumours found in my gullet hence main reason why I found it hard to swallow or drink) and the Cancer had travelled to my stomach.

This was on top of my other illnesses, for example hypertension, high blood pressure, fatty liver, etc. but when one is enjoying life, with a few good drinks, plenty of curry chicken and other real tasty Asian dishes, being 175 cm height but weighing in at 98.8 kg—not forgetting XXL size clothes I wore like 42-44 inch waist trousers—one does not worry ~ until it hits you which is normally too late, in my case it was "in the nick of time".

I had not expected to live after this major operation and the very harsh radiation treatment combined with chemotherapy that followed for two plus months. So it was God's plan for me to survive and "share" my personal journey of despair & hope.

I share with you my own story of my life by the grace of God and let my family (and others) know it is ok to cry and Grown Men can also Cry. It is part of life and part of God's plan.

An arrow can only be shot by pulling it backward.
When life is dragging you back with difficulties, just imagine that it's going to launch you into something great.

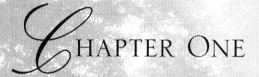

CHAPTER ONE

*The Journey of finding God and
the trip to the Holy Land that
was never to be*

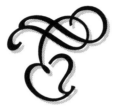

*The Journey of finding God and
the trip to the Holy Land that
was never to be.*

I was never a church-going person. In my younger years I
would go to Sunday school only to receive a free meal and
a chance of getting some nice second-hand clothes to wear.

The church we went to in Cambridge (outside London,
UK) was the Church of England, but like I said I never felt any
belonging to the Church. Our family was very poor and we lived
in the countryside working on farms. We would go from farm to
farm looking for work and from school to school too whenever
school fees or new textbooks or uniforms were required in order
get away from paying for any.

Even during my adult life and during my 20 years in the
New Zealand Army, never did I ever feel the need for God as
I considered myself to be one of the black sheep whenever the
subject of Church came up.

When I was in my early 20s, I married Maggie. I met her during my posting in Singapore in the late 1970s. We lived in New Zealand and had three children—Shaun (who has now changed his name to Chris), Sharon and Shane. After almost 20 years of marriage, we returned to Singapore, separated and both of us remarried. I married Karen in 2001 and we had a daughter Michelle in 2003.

The challenge of accepting the faith was compounded by the fact that Karen is a cradle Catholic, and my mother-in-law, being a staunch Christian woman—who attends so many churches and belongs to so many church groups—saw that it was her mission to "enlighten" me about God and the wonders of his grace and being.

There were times when I could sense a sadness in my wife. We did not have a Church wedding, and when we lived in Choa Chu Kang, she would go to Church by herself and subsequently bring Michelle with her. She told me that Michelle (who was then age 4 or 5) had asked "Why does Daddy not come with us to Church?" I had always thought it best to let my children follow their own path when it comes to Church as long as they leave me out of it. But of course my daughter at that age was so direct and so innocent, little did she know that she had planted a seed in my mind which had started to grow and began to make me question what going to church really meant for my wife and Michelle.

It was not until 2006 that my wife asked "Why not come to Church of the Risen Christ (a Catholic Church) for a talk on Wednesday evening and we have supper afterwards?" My mother-in-law had a plan and she had nudged my wife into persuading me. I agreed to attend for just that one night for the sake of my wife and Michelle, and to see and hear for myself.

On arriving I was asked to fill out a form, and I joined a group of about 10 people; there were around 7 to 8 groups being formed. In the group there were seven of our family members, hence I was outnumbered from the start. But I found the discussion quite interesting and questioned a number of issues (being the black sheep I was) and after a few hours we all left and our small group of family members went for supper. I thought this was the beginning and end of it, little did I know there was a plan for me. Yes, God's plan was put in motion.

"Weeping may endure for a night, but joy
cometh in the morning."—Psalms 30:5

It was not until the following Wednesday that I found out that we were going again to the same Church and for a group discussion, I asked my wife "Why do I need to attend again, and was told "My dear, don't you know you signed up for a 12-month RCIA course so you can learn all about God, the Catholic Church and after finishing the 12 months, you can be baptised and become a real Catholic and member of the Catholic faith." RCIA is the acronym for Rite of Christian Initiation for Adults.

I was stunned, shocked and at a loss for words. I was not angry or upset; just filled with the emotional impact of overwhelming events. So I just continued to attend the sessions and as the weeks went by I found the discussions more and more interesting. I was challenging people and their statements, and the passages of the Bible; I clung onto the belief that "seeing is always believing". Yet the more questions I asked, the more people were willing to explain to me.

I began to look forward to our weekly RCIA meetings and discussions and over the months, one person stood out and was always willing to listen and give advice from her heart. And over time I realised that God had sent an Angel to me and her name was Irene—one of the organisers (support group) for the RCIA course. I had also met other really nice people including my Godpa Raymund who to this day is always around to support me. There was also my good friend Bill who turned out to be very blessed and touched by God's word and we are very much committed in doing God's work for the poor in the Philippines and are actively seeking ways to this day to turn this belief and desire into reality with God's blessing, hopefully sometime soon.

2007 was an unforgettable year. My father-in-law (Karen's dad) passed away in February, and my son who was living in New Zealand was diagnosed with Cancer. Karen, Michelle and I took a trip to New Zealand and were glad to hear that the operation had gone smoothly.

I was baptised in May 2007. Since that big day, I had felt for the first time in my life that there was truly a God and that he is watching over us and will reveal his plan "in his time".

We (Karen, Michelle and mother-in-law Cecilia) went on a number of church outings to Malaysia. We went on a coach tour with a Church Group called *Café*. (Mid-2007 this group was renamed *F.R.E.E.* which stands for Faith, Renewal, Exploration & Evangelisation under Church of the Risen Christ; I joined as Treasurer and my wife joined as Head of Publicity then. To this day, we continue to participate in the meetings and gatherings). I found out so much about the Church and the Miracles that have happened to so many believers, this inspired a desire in me to go to the Holy land, to Israel, Jordon and Egypt and we (Karen and I) often talked about that day when our finances would allow us both to do a Pilgrimage together. My wife has travelled all over the world but one of the few places she has never been to was to the Holy land, and when I joined the Catholic Church the desire grew even more strongly.

Then one day in mid-2010, my mother-in-law surprised us when she signed both Karen and I up for a church group tour including her brother Uncle Tony and his wife Leena for a December 2010 trip to the Holy land. We were so happy and excited. The Spiritual Director of the trip was Father Paul Staes who had blessed us at our wedding. We gave thanks to the Lord for this plan to happen, tickets were purchased, money was changed to local currency, things were all being packed and ready for the trip, and enquiries were made for travel insurance just a few weeks before departure, so we were counting down the weeks and days to the big event.

As I was having some issues with what I thought was heartburn and feeling a bit sick with tummy upsets and I started to find it difficult to swallow 'hard' food like meats, etc., I decided to get myself checked out by the local clinic (Toa Payoh Polyclinic) just in case I needed some medication to bring along with me during the Middle East trip. After seeing the doctor I was told I had reflux and he gave me some pills and said to take these for 2 weeks and if there was no improvement, to come back for another appointment. Well there was no improvement and two weeks later, I felt in fact that it had gotten worse. I went back and got examined by another doctor and got told the same story which I refused to accept. I asked for a referral to the hospital for a more detailed check-up and by chance got an appointment within a few days at Tan Tock Seng Hospital (TTSH).

The day came for the appointment. After waiting for over 3 hours (must be standard procedure for hospitals to keep people waiting for hours even after your appointment time) I went in not knowing what to expect. After some prods and pokes and questions, I was told I would need to have an endoscopy and seeing I had plans to go overseas within the next 2 weeks the doctor had made a request for this to be done as an "Urgent" case. Sure enough the endoscopy appointment was made and confirmed within days (I was getting amazed how efficient things were happening . . . very unlike Government hospitals). Now if you never had an endoscopy before, then let me explain—they put a tube inside you with a camera attached and claws to take samples of whatever is inside so they can run tests to help determine what the problem was. Now there's only two ways of inserting this long tube, one is via your mouth and the other one is at the opposite end of your body . . .

So here I was about to enter into the unknown, no pre-op gown needed just say "Arrrh" and they spray your mouth to numb the area, giving you something to knock you out but before you go into dreamland they insert this plastic mouth guard and stick this darn long tube down your throat and you quickly realise how a drowning person feels fighting for breath, then you are 'knocked out'.

One should not wake up until 30-45 minutes "after" the procedure where they offer you a Milo drink and crackers but in my case I woke up half-way through the procedure only to be inches away from a TV screen showing my very own "insides" which the surgeon was using to determine what portions of tissue he wanted to cut away for samples. And I was quite calmly saying to myself "Wow cool man" and I remember the surgeon say "almost done, don't worry" then I was knocked out again (I guess the amount of drugs they had to put me under was not calculated correctly for a large-sized westerner like me weighing in at almost 100 kg; most Asians are small-sized around half my body weight and mass). Easy to say I survived that ordeal but from then on, each time I go for an endoscopy I always ask for a double dose to "really" knock me out proper.

Another surprise was being called in to review my results within a few days. My son Shane and my wife Karen was with me. We were the last patients for Dr Christopher. It was about 4.30pm and we had waited at least an hour. Dr Chris had bad news. It was Cancer.

"Be strong and of good courage, fear not, nor be afraid . . . for the Lord thy God, he it is that doth go with thee; he will not fail thee, nor forsake thee."
—Deuteronomy 31:6

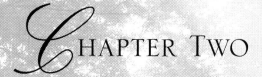

CHAPTER TWO

Options—To Do or Not to Do

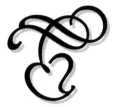

Options—To Do or Not to Do . . .

Okay. At a time like this, what does one say? Let alone think? I had to act fast.

"What are my options?" I asked.

Dr Chris asked instead if we needed time, as a family, to have a few moments. He said it is normal when they tell someone news of this nature, they need time to take it all in.

I had to find my mask. Where is it? All these years of being able to hide my emotions by wearing my mask . . . Where is it now? My mind was racing, then suddenly I found myself and turned to my wife, gave her half a smile and holding back my tears, I held her hand.

I wanted to know what the next steps were. Dr Chris said I would need to see a surgeon to discuss what my options were.

Dr Chris thought I looked very calm. "Well," I said, "must have been the 20 years of Army training." But inside of me,

I knew it was the magic of my mask and maybe God's way of protecting my family, and allowing me to cope.

I walked out stunned even though I knew my mask was still in place, it was like having an out of body experience. I went out to the counter, and again everything went like clockwork and I had an appointment with the Specialist Surgeon in a few days.

I could see myself walking, holding my wife's hand, and stopping to ask where was Shane (my youngest son). My wife replied he was waiting outside in the corridor. So again I could see myself from above walking to talk to my son to discuss the bad news.

As I came in front of my son I could feel myself coming down from above and entering my body once more. There I stood trying to speak and find the words to give him comfort at the same time. It was at this point reality set in and the knowledge that I had just been told I had advanced stage Cancer. My mind was racing but my movements and actions were slow.

I just gave him a hug and heard myself say "I have Cancer and need an urgent operation, don't worry Karen will look after you." His reply was also quiet and he said OK . . . maybe his studies in Radiography prepared him for all types of life threatening illnesses but his quietness told volumes that he was also taken aback.

We contacted my daughter Sharon and arranged to meet her at Novena Square shopping centre, at Harry's, a small Pub (just love the Irish beer) around 7pm. So when we arrived I ordered my Kilkenny Beer and soon afterwards Sharon turned up and I bought the same for her. Then I said I have some important news to share with her and explained briefly what the doctors just told me few hours before and what to expect. Sharon was shocked, tears rolling down her cheeks and we held hands for support.

During the short time spent together we all found it hard to be talkative and only had one drink and some small snacks to eat and decided to go home early.

The ride home which was only 10 minutes away seemed like forever, until this day I cannot remember anyone speaking to each other during this long drive home. I think we were all in a state of shock.

It was now only a few days before our intended overseas trip. We were again at the hospital and told to wait for the doctor. This time my mother-in-law was with us. When we went in, a sober looking middle-aged doctor glazed over my report, asked us to wait as he got the Senior Surgeon (Dr Rao) to join him and now there were two of them looking sober and glazed over the report. Then time slowed down like slow motion as Dr Rao explained they had found 3 tumours and the sample tissues taken had confirmed it was Cancer, yes the Big C.

Again I asked for the truth the whole truth and nothing but the truth—what was my survival rate and if I could still go on my trip to the Holy Land. Again I could hear the answers in slow motion and it was made quite clear I could NOT go on any trip as my condition was very serious and needed urgent medical attention.

We discussed various options, most were not viable other than surgery. One could, of course seek another medical opinion, do more tests and be back at square one, or one could be in denial and believe all this was a bad joke and the doctors don't really know what's going on and go on the 2 weeks' trip hoping that some off-the-counter medicine purchased at a local pharmacy be it in Singapore or in the Middle East, would make this heartburn go away. Or ask now for some strong antibiotics to be prescribed and somehow work. My mind was racing and while the doctors were thinking of what to say, I was also thinking . . . but now no longer in slow motion but in fast forward.

Then suddenly I came to a conclusion—let's go for the Operation now, no need to wait. I want it over and done with. Again I could see the shock in the doctor's eyes, don't I need time to consider was the reply. NO was my answer. If it needs to be done then why wait? I am prepared for anything (but in reality I was very ill-prepared and was about to embark on a journey of my lifetime).

After making my decision to go ahead with the Operation, I asked again for more details of what to expect; the Who, What, Why and When. On the Who, the surgeon's team would be both doctors seated in front of me, one of them was Snr Surgeon Dr Rao. It was to be approximately a 4- to 5-hour procedure to operate on my oesophagus and stomach and what they find will determine the extent of the next phase (to try and save as much of the stomach as possible). They will make a small incision in my back (turned out to be the largest incision ever) to assist in the removal of the tumours (they took out the gallbladder too as I was told I had a number of large gallstones, like a special reward for making up your mind straightaway you get a free removal service . . .).

Then within 1-2 weeks I would be able to leave the hospital and start my other treatment (which was to be Radiation and Chemo—but details of this kept quiet so as not to overwhelm me with all this wonderful news). How easy all this sounds, all over within 1-2 weeks. Hmmm, if only it turned out that way.

The doctors said that a number of scans would be required, (well that was downplayed as I had a number of X Rays, CT Scans, MRI Scan, talk about feeling like being placed inside of a microwave), still all these were required to pin-point where the

Cancer is and to what extent, that said they will only know for certain after "opening me up" . . .

We needed to sign up for Admission to the hospital and Karen happened to see one of her clients, Lynn, who had been recently posted to the Admissions department (Karen had written advertorials for the hospital on their wellness programmes). Lynn gave us some good advice on TTSH and the procedures, and to our surprise she mentioned that Dr Rao is one of the most senior surgeons in his field and gave us additional assurance that he would personally take charge of my well-being and I should consider myself to be very lucky (as luck would have it he turned out to be very good apart from a small hiccup during the operation of which I will enlighten you all later). So I was to be in good hands.

Over the next few days we continued to discuss what our options were, if we should get a second opinion, use different methods of treatment, etc. We got so many conflicting quick fix remedies, stories of miracles were related to us, and we were bombarded with alternative medication from Chinese to Western herbal treatments, most I would say came from the vast internet and some from well-wishes from friends and Church people I know and many I did not know. All this was more overwhelming to me than the actual day the doctors told me the news; how strange it was to get more upset by well-wishers than by getting the news of the Big C direct!

Karen had to quit teaching her classes at the enrichment centre. She informed her clients and close friends what had happened, and that she would work from home in order to help me during my recovery (My wife had turned out to be my pillar of strength). Tati, our helper from Indonesia, turned out to be a great help too, during this period.

I remember wanting to go to Church and asking God: Why me Lord? What have I done to suffer so much pain? What is your Plan for me? It was not an easy task to do considering I had only just joined the Catholic Church. All this praying and having a relationship with God at this point was somewhat new to me and I kept asking: Why me? Why am I suffering? Why . . . why . . . why?

I realised then I was chosen and the first step was to have faith in Jesus. The choice that I had was to either be angry at God or accept his doing as it is part of his plan for me to suffer, so with tears in my eyes I just accepted his plan and whatever will be will be.

> *"And we know that in all things God works for the good of those who love Him, who have been called according to his purpose."*
> —Romans 8:28

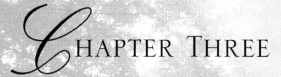

CHAPTER THREE

What is Cancer?—The Big C

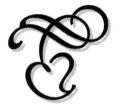

What is Cancer?—The Big C

I had been diagnosed with Oesophageal Cancer where there were 3 tumours in my gullet and the Cancer had spread to my stomach, hence the need to have surgery in two places to remove the affected areas.

To better understand what Oesophageal Cancer is all about, this chapter will provide a quick snapshot about Cancer. Below is information available from the American Cancer Society website (www.cancer.org).

What is Cancer?

Cancer is the general name for a group of more than 100 diseases. Although there are many kinds of cancer, all cancers start because abnormal cells grow out of control. Untreated cancers can cause serious illness and death.

Normal cells in the body

The body is made up of trillions of living cells. Normal body cells grow, divide, and die in an orderly fashion. During the early years of a person's life, normal cells divide faster to allow the person to grow. After the person becomes an adult, most cells divide only to replace worn-out or dying cells or to repair injuries.

How cancer starts

Cancer starts when cells in a part of the body start to grow out of control. Cancer cell growth is different from normal cell growth. Instead of dying, cancer cells continue to grow and form new, abnormal cells. Cancer cells can also invade (grow into) other tissues, something that normal cells cannot do. Growing out of control and invading other tissues are what makes a cell a cancer cell.

Cells become cancer cells because of DNA (deoxyribonucleic acid) damage. DNA is in every cell and it directs all the cell's actions. In a normal cell, when DNA gets damaged the cell either repairs the damage or the cell dies. In cancer cells, the damaged DNA is not repaired, and the cell doesn't die like it should. Instead, the cell goes on making new cells that the body doesn't need. These new cells all have the same abnormal DNA as the first cell does.

People can inherit abnormal DNA, but most DNA damage is caused by mistakes that happen while the normal cell is reproducing or by something in the environment. Sometimes the cause of the DNA damage may be something obvious like cigarette smoking or sun exposure. But it's rare to know exactly what caused any one person's cancer.

In most cases, the cancer cells form a tumour. Some cancers, like leukaemia, rarely form tumours. Instead, these cancer cells involve the blood and blood-forming organs and circulate through other tissues where they grow.

How cancer spreads

Cancer cells often travel to other parts of the body where they begin to grow and form new tumours. This happens when the cancer cells get into the body's bloodstream or lymph vessels. Over time, the tumours replace normal tissue. The process of cancer spreading is called *metastasis*.

How cancers differ

No matter where a cancer may spread, it's always named for the place where it started. For example, breast cancer that has spread to the liver is called metastatic breast cancer, not liver cancer. Likewise, prostate cancer that has spread to the bone is called metastatic prostate cancer, not bone cancer.

Different types of cancer can behave very differently. For instance, lung cancer and skin cancer are very different diseases. They grow at different rates and respond to different treatments. This is why people with cancer need treatment that is aimed at their kind of cancer.

Tumours that are not cancer

Not all tumours are cancer. Tumours that aren't cancer are called *benign*. Benign tumours can cause problems—they can grow very large and press on healthy organs and tissues. But they cannot grow into (invade) other tissues. Because they can't invade, they also can't spread to other parts of the body (metastasize). These tumours are almost never life threatening.

How common is cancer?

Half of all men and one-third of all women in the US will develop cancer during their lifetimes.

Today, millions of people are living with cancer or have had cancer. The risk of developing many types of cancer can be reduced by changes in a person's lifestyle, for example, by staying away from tobacco, limiting time in the sun, being physically active and healthy eating.

There are also screening tests that can be done for some types of cancers so they can be found as early as possible—while they are small and before they have spread. In general, the earlier a cancer is found and treated, the better the chances are for living for many years.

The following information on Cancer Staging and Oesophageal Cancer is from the National Cancer Institute (www.cancer.gov)

Cancer Staging

Staging describes the extent or severity of a person's cancer. Knowing the stage of disease helps the doctor plan treatment and estimate the person's prognosis.

Staging is based on knowledge of the way cancer progresses. Cancer cells grow and divide without control or order, and they do not die when they should. As a result, they often form a mass of tissue called a tumor. As a tumor grows, it can invade nearby tissues and organs. Cancer cells can also break away from a tumor and enter the bloodstream or the lymphatic system. By moving through the bloodstream or lymphatic system, cancer cells can spread from the primary site to lymph nodes or to other organs, where they may form new tumors. The spread of cancer is called metastasis.

Stage	Definition
Stage 0	Carcinoma in situ
Stage I, Stage II, and Stage III	Higher numbers indicate more extensive disease: Larger tumour size and/or spread of the cancer beyond the organ in which it first developed to nearby lymph nodes and/ or tissues or organs adjacent to the location of the primary tumour
Stage IV	The cancer has spread to distant tissues or organs

OESOPHAGEAL CANCER

The Oesophagus

The oesophagus is a muscular tube in the chest. It's about 10 inches (25 cm) long. This organ is part of the digestive tract. Food moves from the mouth through the oesophagus to the stomach.

The wall of the oesophagus has several layers:

- **Inner layer or lining**: The lining (mucosa) of the oesophagus is wet, which helps food to pass to the stomach.
- **Submucosa**: Glands in the submucosa layer make mucus, which helps keep the lining of the oesophagus wet.

- **Muscle layer**: The muscles push food down to the stomach.
- **Outer layer**: The outer layer covers the oesophagus.
  A tumour in the oesophagus can be benign (not cancer) or malignant (cancer):

Benign tumours:

- Are rarely a threat to life
- Don't invade the tissues around them
- Don't spread to other parts of the body
- Can be removed and don't usually grow back

Malignant tumours (cancer of the oesophagus):

- May be a threat to life
- Can invade and damage nearby organs and tissues
- Can spread to other parts of the body
- Sometimes can be removed but may grow back

Oesophageal cancer cells can spread by breaking away from an oesophageal tumour. They can travel through blood vessels or lymph vessels to reach other parts of the body. After spreading, cancer cells may attach to other tissues and grow to form new tumours that may damage those tissues.

When oesophageal cancer spreads from its original place to another part of the body, the new tumour has the same kind of abnormal cells and the same name as the original tumour. For example, if oesophageal cancer spreads to the liver, the cancer cells in the liver are actually oesophageal cancer cells. The disease is metastatic oesophageal cancer, not liver cancer. For that reason, it is treated as cancer of the oesophagus, not liver cancer.

Staging Tests

Staging tests can show the stage (extent) of oesophageal cancer, such as whether cancer cells have spread to other parts of the body. When cancer of the oesophagus spreads, cancer cells are often found in nearby lymph nodes. Oesophageal cancer cells can spread from the oesophagus to almost any other part of the body, such as the liver, lungs, or bones.

Staging tests may include . . .

- **CT scan:** Your doctor may order a CT scan of your chest and abdomen. An x-ray machine linked to a computer will take a series of detailed pictures of these areas. You'll receive contrast material by mouth and by injection into a blood vessel in your arm or hand. The contrast material makes abnormal areas easier to see. The pictures can show cancer that has spread to the liver, lungs, bones, or other organs.
- **PET scan:** Your doctor may use a PET scan to find cancer that has spread. You'll receive an injection of a small amount of radioactive sugar. A machine makes computerized pictures of the sugar being used by cells in the body. Because cancer cells use sugar faster than normal cells, areas with cancer cells look brighter on the pictures. The pictures can show cancer that has spread to the lymph nodes, liver, or other organs.
- **EUS:** A EUS (endoscopic ultrasound) can show how deeply the cancer has invaded the wall of the oesophagus. It can also show whether cancer may have spread to nearby lymph nodes. Your doctor will pass a thin, lighted tube (endoscope) through your mouth to your

oesophagus. A probe at the end of the tube sends out high-energy sound waves. The waves bounce off tissues in your oesophagus and nearby organs, and a computer creates a picture from the echoes. During the exam, the doctor may take tissue samples of lymph nodes.

Stages

Doctors describe the stages of oesophageal cancer using the Roman numerals I, II, III, and IV. Stage I is early-stage cancer, and Stage IV is advanced cancer that has spread to other parts of the body, such as the liver. The stage of cancer of the oesophagus depends mainly on . . .

- How deeply the tumour has invaded the wall of the oesophagus
- The tumour's location (upper, middle, or lower oesophagus)
- Whether oesophageal cancer cells have spread to lymph nodes or other parts of the body

Stages I and II of Adenocarcinoma of the Oesophagus

Stage IA

Cancer has grown through the inner layer and invades the wall of the oesophagus. The grade is 1 or 2.

Stage IB

Cancer has invaded the wall of the oesophagus and is grade 3. Or, cancer has invaded more deeply into the muscle layer of the oesophagus, and the grade is 1 or 2.

Stage IIA

Cancer has invaded the muscle layer of the oesophagus, and the grade is 3.

Stage IIB

Cancer has invaded the outer layer of the oesophagus. Or, cancer has not invaded the outer layer, but cancer cells are also found in one or two nearby lymph nodes.

Stages I and II of Squamous Cell Cancer of the Oesophagus

Stage IA

Cancer has grown through the inner layer and invaded the wall of the oesophagus. The grade is 1.

Stage IB

Cancer has invaded the wall of the oesophagus and is grade 2 or 3. Or, cancer is found in the lower part of the oesophagus, it has invaded the muscle layer or outer layer of the oesophagus, and the grade is 1.

Stage IIA

Cancer is found in the upper or middle part of the oesophagus, it has invaded the muscle layer or outer layer of the oesophagus, and the grade is 1. Or, cancer is found in the lower part of the oesophagus, it has invaded the muscle layer or outer layer of the oesophagus, and the grade is 2 or 3.

Stage IIB

Cancer is found in the upper or middle part of the oesophagus, it has invaded the muscle layer or outer layer of the oesophagus, and the grade is 2 or 3. Or, cancer has not invaded the outer layer, and cancer cells are found in one or two nearby lymph nodes.

Stages III and IV of Oesophageal Cancer (Both Types)

Stage IIIA

Stage IIIA is one of the following:

- Cancer has not invaded the outer layer, and cancer cells are found in 3 to 6 nearby lymph nodes.
- Or, cancer has invaded the outer layer of the oesophagus, and cancer cells are also found in 1 or 2 nearby lymph nodes.

Or, cancer extends through the oesophageal wall and has invaded nearby tissues, such as the <u>diaphragm</u> or <u>pleura</u>. No cancer cells are found in lymph nodes.

Stage IIIB

Cancer has invaded the outer layer of the oesophagus, and cancer cells are found in 3 to 6 nearby lymph nodes.

Stage IIIC

Stage IIIC is one of the following:

- Cancer has invaded tissues near the oesophagus, and cancer cells are found in up to 6 nearby lymph nodes.
- Or, cancer cells are found in 7 or more nearby lymph nodes.

Or, the cancer can't be removed by surgery because the tumor has invaded the <u>trachea</u> or other nearby tissues.

Stage IV

The oesophageal cancer has spread to other parts of the body, such as the liver, lungs, or bones.

Stages of Oesophageal Cancer	Characteristics	Relative 5 Year Survival Rate (%)
0	Cancerous cells are confined to the inner most layer or epithelium	70
I	Cancerous cells invasion goes beyond the epithelium to the submucosa	60
II A	The cells spread further, invading the muscle layer of the oesophagus, and most probably even the adventitia	40
II B	The cells spread beyond the epithelium, but haven't invaded the adventitia as yet	20
III	The cells have invaded the adventitia and spread further to nearby lymph nodes or even to the nearby organs	15
IV A	The cells have spread to distant lymph nodes	15
IV B	Cancerous cells have spread to distant lymph nodes and/or other organs	Below 5

The survival for Oesophageal Cancer is low.
Source: Cancer Focus, Volume 10, No. 4, 2010, Singapore Cancer Society.

Treatment

People with cancer of the oesophagus have many treatment options. Treatment options include . . .

- Surgery
- Radiation Therapy
- Chemotherapy
- Targeted Therapy

Surgery

Surgery may be an option for people with early-stage cancer of the oesophagus. Usually, the surgeon removes the section of the oesophagus with the cancer, a small amount of normal tissue around the cancer, and nearby lymph nodes. Sometimes, part or all of the stomach is also removed.

If only a very small part of the stomach is removed, the surgeon usually reshapes the remaining part of the stomach into a tube and joins the stomach tube to the remaining part of the oesophagus in the neck or chest. Or, a piece of large intestine or small intestine may be used to connect the stomach to the remaining part of the oesophagus.

If the entire stomach needs to be removed, the surgeon will use a piece of intestine to join the remaining part of the oesophagus to the small intestine.

During surgery, the surgeon may place a feeding tube into your small intestine. This tube helps you get enough nutrition while you heal.

You may have pain from the surgery. However, your health care team will give you medicine to help control the pain. Before surgery, you may want to discuss the plan for pain relief with your health care team. After surgery, they can adjust the plan if you need more pain relief.

Your health care team will watch for pneumonia or other infections, breathing problems, bleeding, food leaking into the chest, or other problems that may require treatment.

The time it takes to heal after surgery is different for everyone. Your hospital stay may be a week or longer, and your recovery will continue after you leave the hospital.

Radiation Therapy

Radiation therapy is an option for people with any stage of oesophageal cancer. The treatment affects cells only in the area being treated, such as the throat and chest area.

Radiation therapy may be given before, after, or instead of surgery. Chemotherapy is usually given along with radiation therapy.

Radiation therapy for oesophageal cancer may be given to . . .

- Destroy the cancer
- Help shrink the tumour so that you can swallow more easily
- Help relieve pain from cancer that has spread to bone or other tissues

Doctors use two types of radiation therapy to treat oesophageal cancer. Some people receive both types:

- **Machine outside the body**: The radiation comes from a large machine. This is called external radiation therapy. The machine aims radiation at your body to kill cancer cells. It doesn't hurt. You'll go to a hospital or clinic, and you'll lie down on a treatment table. Each treatment session usually lasts less than 20 minutes. Treatments are usually given 5 days a week for several weeks.
- **Radioactive material inside the body** (brachytherapy): The doctor numbs your throat with an anaesthetic spray

and gives you medicine to help you relax. The doctor puts a tube into your oesophagus. The radiation comes from the tube. After the tube is removed, no radioactivity is left in your body. Usually, one treatment session is needed. Because the treatment session lasts one to two days, you'll probably stay in a special room at the hospital.

The side effects of radiation therapy depend mainly on the type of radiation therapy, how much radiation is given, and the part of your body that is treated.

External radiation therapy aimed at the chest may cause a sore throat, cough, or shortness of breath. You may feel a lump in your throat or burning in your chest or throat when you swallow. After several weeks of treatment, it may be painful to swallow. Your health care team can suggest ways to manage these problems. The problems usually go away when treatment ends.

External radiation therapy can harm the skin. It's common for the skin in the chest area to become red and dry and to get darker. Sometimes the skin may feel tender or itchy. Check with your doctor before using lotion or cream on your chest. After treatment is over, the skin will heal.

You're likely to become tired during external radiation therapy, especially in the later weeks of treatment. Although getting enough rest is important, most people say they feel better when they exercise every day. Try to go for a short walk, do gentle stretches, or do yoga.

Years after either type of radiation therapy, the oesophagus may become narrow. If this happens, it may feel like food is getting stuck in your chest. Usually, a gastroenterologist can treat this problem.

Chemotherapy

Most people with oesophageal cancer get chemotherapy. It may be used alone or with radiation therapy.

Chemotherapy uses drugs to kill cancer cells. The drugs for cancer of the oesophagus are usually given directly into a vein (intravenously) through a thin needle.

You'll probably receive chemotherapy in a clinic or at the doctor's office. People rarely need to stay in the hospital during treatment.

The side effects depend mainly on the drugs given and amount of chemotherapy that you get. Chemotherapy kills fast-growing cancer cells, but the drugs can also harm normal cells that divide rapidly:

- Blood cells: When drugs lower the levels of healthy blood cells, you're more likely to get infections, bruise or bleed easily, and feel very weak and tired. Your health care team will check for low levels of blood cells. If your levels are low, your health care team may stop the chemotherapy for a while or reduce the dose of the drug. They may also give you medicines that help your body to make new blood cells.

- Cells in hair roots: Chemotherapy may cause hair loss. If you lose your hair, it will grow back after treatment, but the colour and texture may be changed.

- Cells that line the digestive tract: Chemotherapy can cause a poor appetite, nausea and vomiting, diarrhoea, or mouth and lip sores. Your healthcare team can give you medicines and suggest other ways to help with these problems.

Other possible side effects include a skin rash, joint pain, tingling or numbness in your hands and feet, hearing problems, or swollen feet or legs.

When radiation therapy and chemotherapy are given at the same time, the side effects may be worse.

Your healthcare team can suggest ways to control many of these problems. Most go away when treatment ends.

Targeted Therapy

People with oesophageal cancer that has spread may receive a type of treatment called targeted therapy. This treatment can block the growth and spread of oesophageal cancer cells.

Targeted therapy for cancer of the oesophagus is usually given intravenously. The treatment enters the bloodstream and can affect cancer cells all over the body.

During treatment, your health care team will watch you for side effects. You may get diarrhoea, belly pain, heartburn, joint pain, tingling arms and legs, or heart problems. Most side effects usually go away after treatment ends.

Nutrition

It's important for you to be well nourished before, during, and after cancer treatment. Being well nourished may help you feel better, have more energy, and get the most benefit from your treatment.

However, oesophageal cancer and its treatment can make it hard to be well nourished, and it may be hard for you to not lose weight. For many reasons, you may not feel like eating. For example, you may have nausea or trouble swallowing, and the foods you used to like to eat could now cause discomfort.

If you're unable to eat, special treatments or other ways of getting nutrition may be needed. If the cancer in your oesophagus makes it very hard to swallow food, your health care team may suggest that you have radiation therapy to shrink the tumour. Or, they may suggest that a plastic or metal mesh tube (stent) be put in your oesophagus to keep it open. Another option is for you to receive nutrition through a feeding tube. Sometimes, intravenous nutrition is needed.

Nutrition After Surgery

If your stomach is removed during surgery for oesophageal cancer, you may develop dumping syndrome. After meals, people with dumping syndrome may have cramps, nausea, bloating, diarrhoea, and dizziness.

If you have dumping syndrome, a registered dietician can help you learn how to be well nourished without making your symptoms worse. Here are some tips for preventing or controlling the symptoms of dumping syndrome:

- Try to eat at least 6 small meals each day.
- Sit up during meals and for at least 30 minutes afterward.
- Chew food very well.
- Eat mostly solid meals, and drink liquids between meals.
- Avoid very sweet foods and drinks.
- After surgery, ask your health care team whether you need a dietary supplement, such as calcium or vitamin B12.

Follow-Up Care

You'll need regular check-ups (such as every 3 to 6 months) after treatment for cancer of the oesophagus. Check-ups help ensure that any changes in your health are noted and treated if needed. If you have any health problems between check-ups, contact your doctor.

Cancer of the oesophagus may come back after treatment. Your doctor will check for the return of cancer. It may return in the chest or it may return in another part of the body, such as the liver.

Check-ups also help detect health problems that can result from cancer treatment.

Check-ups may include a physical exam, blood tests, chest x-rays, CT scans, endoscopy, or other tests.

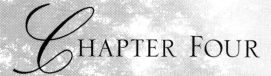

CHAPTER FOUR

Let the Battle begin—
bring it on

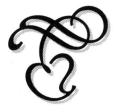

Let the Battle begin—bring it on

Must be my Army training and 20 years of experience kicking in, I wanted to fight this Cancer head-on no matter what, even if I was unsure of what to expect. We contacted a few friends who had Cancer and they tried to give us some insight on how they coped, but Cancer affects different people in different ways and me having what you might say a double dose of cancer (Oesophageal & Stomach) on top of Hypertension, High Blood Pressure, Fatty Liver and what other illnesses untold or unknown to me; I knew my fight would not be easy, but the saying goes, *"Once a Soldier Always a Soldier",* so let the battle begin.

> *"In his heart a man plans his course,*
> *But the LORD determines his steps."*
> —Proverbs 16:9

It was not an easy task to decide what to do as I was still not sure as to what to expect during the treatments, and what the chances would be. All I knew was I was about to go through a life-changing personal experience which would make me a different person.

This was a life and death decision and I was extremely concerned. Do I have the right to decide this all by myself? What about my loved ones, do they have a right to decide for me? Whichever route I took, not only would my life be affected but my whole family would suffer the brunt of it as well.

I decided to fight this illness head-on and for the sake of my family I would get all the finances in order and a Will to be arranged just in case. I learnt a hard lesson seeing my Father-in-law pass away within a few weeks of getting ill and leaving a mess for my Mother-in-law as the bank accounts, properties, etc. were not in joint names, so you can imagine the hassle of just drawing a small amount of funds to live off, let alone large amounts of investments and properties not in her name. So I was determined not to put my wife and family in the same situation.

I spent hours sorting out all the documents, where our investments were, made joint bank accounts and typed out a long list explaining what, where and how to find and account for everything. Then came the Will, what to do for my wife and my four children. This was hard to do knowing that in a few days I would be under the knife. Then surviving that I had to go through radiation plus chemo treatment, but I was focused on not leaving a mess for my wife to sort out if I did not make it.

So the Will was drafted up, even my wife made her own Will (two for the price of one . . . special discount by the lawyer) and made the appointment with the Company lawyer, only to be told I could not sign it as I was "Not in the right frame of mind". What rubbish was this . . . I told him I was at peace with what was about to happen and I wish to ensure if I pass away my family would be taken care of, hence I consider myself to be in the right frame of mind. So to overcome this issue I had to get someone to "certify" that I am in the right frame of mind and that I know what I am doing and fully aware that I am about to undergo a major operation for Cancer, only then was I able to sign my own Will and have it counter-signed and stamped by the lawyer. The lesson here is "not" to wait for the last minute when you are ill to write up your Will.

We went to several healing masses at Church and was prayed over many times. I found myself on an entirely different faith level. I felt ashamed that I was not able to be as devoted to God and have as much faith in the Lord as my Brothers and Sisters in Christ had and whom were all willing to pray over me and asking God to protect and heal me. What would happen to me if I were to be prayed over and not get healed? What right did I have to question God? I had even asked our Parish Priest Fr John Sim for an anointing to bless and prepare me in my sickness.

(Anointment is used to endow an ordinary person with special holiness. In the Roman Catholic Church, unction was long regarded as a last rite, usually postponed until death was imminent and the dying Christian was *in extremis;* thus, the name extreme unction developed. In modern times, a more lenient interpretation permitted anointing of the less seriously ill).[1]

This was my very first holy anointment and I did not know what to expect, but the grace of God touched me and I felt a

---

[1]   http://www.britannica.com/EBchecked/topic/26542/anointment

glow inside of me; I believed it was the Holy Spirit protecting me and giving me strength to carry on the good fight.

I felt I needed to suffer and go through this painful process in order to understand God's plan for me and appreciate his work, and just maybe my sharing and writing of this book is his plan so that others can share and understand that it is ok for *Grown Men to Cry* and to trust others.

So vulnerable and frightened I was. One might use laughter and comedy to ward off the tears, (laughter could make almost any situation tolerable), or else you had to learn the art of wearing a mask. So into battle I went, chin up, cracking jokes just to make others laugh and feel better, and not to have the so called "Pity Me" parade.

Then the day finally arrived and so . . . I prayed.

"Father come to me. Hold me up 'cause I can barely stand
My strength is gone and my breath is short,
I can't reach out my hands
But my heart is set on a pilgrimage to heaven's own"

I lay in the hospital bed—dressed in a white operating gown all prepped for the main event of my life—outside the Operating Theatre of Tan Tock Seng Hospital (TTSH) Singapore, located 10 minutes from our home.

I was admitted into TTSH on 28 November 2010, went through all the Pre-Op setup, said my goodbyes, etc. and was wheeled to the Pre-Op room. I waited for almost an hour, only to be told no Intensive Care Unit (ICU) room was available, hence no operation could take place and that I needed to re-schedule the operation.

As mine was a very urgent case, we managed to re-schedule the Operation for 2 December after paying an extra S$3,000 for the ICU room on top of the S$8,000 deposit for the Operation ~ hence the re-run of Pre-Op preparation and the Goodbyes were undertaken a second time, with the repetitive ritual of being asked my name and Singapore identification (i/c) number endless times, being asked endless times if I had fasted (not eaten for at least 8 hours) and briefing me on what was about to happen in the Operating room (in fact very little said so I just blanked things out). Without a doubt this was going to be a major surgery. The surgeons would be removing part of my gullet as well as my stomach. After the operation, I learnt they took out my gallbladder too.

Then along came a Nurse, "Hi Mr Robert," (They always get my name wrong, using my surname as my first name, grr . . .) "how are we today . . . . (Now why would anyone ask such a question when you are literally lying in wait outside an Operation room?) Then came the quiz—What's your name? What's your i/c number? You know why you are here? And so on. It's normal practice to check and double check your details but the Nurse had only really needed to check my wrist band for the details Anyway I played along and answered all her questions, must have been the 6th or 7th time I was asked that day.

Next came the scary stuff . . .

I was wheeled into the Operating theatre. Lights, camera, action . . . It flashed through my mind that this was just like it was in the movies: the lights shining down on you, all the people inside wearing their masks and gowns, and there it was—right in the middle of the room was the long plain-looking operating table. Somehow it reminded me of a dentist chair. Then, like a swarm of ants, all these people came over to me, some asking my name and i/c number, some asking me to roll over so they could lift me onto the operating table. I remember one of them, must have been the Senior Surgeon, giving me some assurance that he would do his best and not to worry. Then came the plastic mask, and I could feel my heart pumping faster and faster, finding it harder to breathe and suddenly I was out.

About five hours later I was in the recovery room waiting to be stabilised before going to the Intensive Care Unit (ICU). It seemed like forever before I woke up in this small room with all these tubes inside of me (at least eight or nine). It felt like the doctors had inserted foreign objects into all the natural holes created by God, and where there were no holes, they would create one.

I would see people inside my room but not know who they were (they were actually family members). I would drift in and out of consciousness and it would take a few days more before I could make out who was who.

I was told that I had muttered a few works like "It's painful" and was groaning most of the time. I was unable to move or lift my arms. In fact I scared the nurse assigned to me as my heart stopped 3 or 4 times. To me, I was so drugged up I didn't have a care in the world but seeing this very young nurse (looked to be in her twenties only) panicking over me just made me chuckle inside.

Every few hours another nurse would come in and give me a range of injections 4 to 5 at a time, mostly through the four tubes in my neck and 1 or 2 in my hand or arm or stomach area; I was like a pin cushion.

I barely remember my good friend Roy visiting me in the ICU (somehow he got past the hospital guards and nurses, and just walked in). He was shocked to see me with all the tubes and monitors connected to me.

After four days in the ICU, I was moved to my hospital room. We had booked a private room with air-conditioning, not that we were well off but I must have my air-con as the nights would be 25+ degrees C here in Singapore and this Kiwi guy just needs his air-con at night to sleep. This came with a high price tag but comfort and recovery were first priority.

The time came when I was moved from the ICU to the top floor A Class ward where my wife met me and the handover from the ICU staff to the A Class Nurse was done. According to my wife, the Staff Nurse flipped out asking why the patient was being transferred to her ward where clearly he had one too many tubes and needed 24-hour watch over him with heart monitors, etc. which the ward was not equipped with, let alone prepared to cope with such an extremely ill patient, or words to that effect . . . As for me I was in wonderland, having been pumped with morphine and other pain-killing drugs. If you left me in the corridor, I wouldn't have complained unless my morphine ran out then I would be in trouble.

Anyway when I came to, I was all alone in a strange room on a strange bed with a TV switched on facing me. I believe it was on a Chinese Channel. How perceptive and caring towards this Westerner. Then there were faces appearing, am I in heaven? But slowly the faces would turn out to be family members trying to talk to me and I would just groan "Oh the pain . . ."

Hours turned into days and days turned into weeks. As time went by, I was starting to feel the effects of the operation. Each day, morning and night, a whole team of doctors would come into my room, look at my chart and leave. It wasn't until the second week that I had enough strength to ask some questions like "How did it go? What did you do? What was the outcome? Did you get all the Cancer affected areas?" Strangely as I asked each doctor more questions as the days went by, I would find out more and more things from them. Maybe they had wanted to keep some things from me or thought I was perhaps not strong enough to hear the truth, but in my case I just wanted to know.

My wife would usually stay with me most of the night, returning home at 2 to 3am in the morning. As the days went by, I grew stronger but was not able to eat until the third week. I was having daily x-rays and sometimes two x-rays in the same day. What was strange was that most of them were conducted in my room with a portable x-ray machine, but on a few occasions I had to be transported, tubes and all, down to the x-ray room. Later, when examining the hospital bill, we realised that the portable x-rays cost a lot more too. On one occasion, I was asked to get up from my wheelchair, walk over and lie down on the x-ray table. I had to tell her I could not stand, let alone walk with all these tubes connected to me.

Seems this person was not informed that I had just undergone a major surgery. She was determined to order me to stand up, and when I repeated myself, she walked away and in an angry voice, she complained to another person who in turn went outside and brought yet another person into the room (must had been her senior?). After explaining to him what I just went through, he immediately understood my situation and told this junior person not to conduct the x-ray as it will be done later in my room.

Every day they would take blood samples and I was convinced I was a real live dummy for new doctors to practise drawing blood; my hands were black and blue—both of them—and I would shudder at the very thought that it was time yet again to donate my blood for daily tests.

Also a daily event was the changing of my bedsheets. It would take 2 to 3 nurses and sometimes my wife to help lift me and move me in order to take away the sheets and replace them with clean ones. I had to inject an extra dose of morphine 10 minutes before this epic event. Ideally I had to start moving so as not to have bed sores, but how was I to move? I had a major operation on my stomach, a major operation on my back, tubes in the left side of me, tubes in the right side of me, tubes in my back, tubes in my neck, tubes in my hands, tubes in my nose and even in my "little" one . . . how to move? And even when I did get shifted, I was not at all comfortable.

One day I complained that my back felt sore, as well as hot and wet. It was not until two nurses bent me forward and lifted my shirt did they discover that the skin on my back was splitting, literally coming apart, and the hot and wetness was me bleeding. Again flashback to seeing the nurses panic at the ICU, but this time I was aware of what was happening. So they "taped" me up, changed the sheets and pumped some more antibiotics into me (I was taking 4 different antibiotics, pumped daily and directly into my neck via the tubes inserted).

The days went by and the nights were long, and I had many hours to think and to pray to God. I would ask for forgiveness and pray that the Lord give strength to my family and loved ones. And in time, for my pain to be reduced so that I could fight the good fight.

I had to start breathing exercises every hour as one of my lungs had been collapsed during surgery. At one point they suspected I might have lung infection or pneumonia. Anyway I needed to exercise my lungs by blowing into this plastic tube to get a reading. At first I was told to try to get to level 40 and after my second day during one of the doctor's visits the doctor asked me if I was doing my breathing exercises, I proudly said "Yes, I can now reach 40", in which his reply was "Only 40? You should be doing 100!" Oh what a disappointment I felt, but I soldiered on and as each day passed I made improvements; even in the middle of the night I would try this exercise. It's what saved me from the lung infection and made possible my recovery from the collapsed lung, otherwise I may not have made it.

I would look forward to the many visits from my family and their friends and even Church people I'd never met. I even missed seeing my mother-in-law as she went on the trip to the Holy Land on our tickets so as not to waste them, even though she had been there 3 times before. Still what could I do? Here I was flat on my back in hospital, lucky to be alive. The Middle East Holy Land trip will happen another day, I am sure of it, it is God's will and in his time.

My youngest daughter Michelle was so amazed by all the medical issues I was having. She would just sit beside my bed, hold my hand or stroke my arm to ease the pain as she could see in my eyes tears forming and that I was unable to talk. My wife would wipe a wet cotton wool over my lips to moisten them, puff up the pillows for me and over time help me sit up and move me around the room and to the toilet. By week three, I was able to stand for short periods and had to start daily exercises. I would just walk around the room for a start, with a walking cane and two people to assist, then down to one and then on my own. The physical exercises were challenging but I also completed what was asked of me and did one extra round to satisfy myself and soon it was time to take on the stairs, well that was easier said than done. In fact I was able to step up 4 steps but when asked to walk down I just broke down and cried. I was so scared of falling I froze and dared not move, it took ages for my wife and physiotherapist to convince me I was ok and that I would not fall down. It was a strange feeling because here I was hobbling around in a wheelchair and on crutches, then with walking aids but when it came to four steps to walk down I froze and started to cry . . .

I remember the day when Chris, my eldest son, had to fly back to New Zealand. I was upset and tried hard to wear my mask and not show it, but I think he knew and gave me a big hug and said "You'll be ok, us Roberts family are fighters." In fact it was only a few years before that Chris had cancer and had a tumour taken out from his stomach the size of a big orange he said, and he had discharged himself from the hospital after three days saying if he had to die he would want to die at home, not in a hospital. In 2007, we went over to New Zealand with Michelle to give our support and help him out the best way we could. So he is right, the Roberts family are fighters and my son has proven this to me as today he still goes for check-ups to make sure he is cancer free.

Sharon, my eldest daughter, would drop by after her work and would sometimes bring her friends with her and we would play a board game or cards. Or if I was too tired, I would watch them play instead, it was enjoyable and helped pass the time, sometimes too quickly.

One thing I could not understand was here I was in hospital after a major operation on my stomach, and of all things visitors would bring fruits, cakes or bird's nest for me to eat and drink. Hey it was only in week two that I was given a straw and allowed to sip a few drops of water let alone eat any food. Strange but it seemed to be the thing to do, maybe they brought not for me but for the visitors who might feel like an orange or kiwifruit or something . . .

Soon I was starting to become a bit more mobile, but I still had all these tubes in me. So the doctors decided that over the next few days they would reduce the number of tubes, starting with the four in my neck which turned out to be the least painful to remove; one quick pull and out came the 2-foot tube and on went the plaster, job done. Then there was the one inserted in my little willy, now this was damn painful and quite embarrassing as a lady doctor did it and again one quick pull, and out from Bob's your Uncle came this long tube, how the hell did they put that inside of me . . .

Now for the tube inserted to the left of my stomach. Seeing there was very little bleeding in the last two weeks, it was decided that it was time to take out that tube too. However this tube was far thicker than the others and the tissue around my reduced stomach had started to grow around the tube—hence I was told this could be a little bit painful, now how do you gauge a little bit? I was told to take a deep breath, and lo and behold the nurse yanked it out in one quick swoop and I yelled out in one loud voice "What the hell!" or words to that effect. I think the whole ward heard me, but I must confess it was damn painful and not just a little bit.

Now what was left was the tube in my right side, I think the nurse was too taken aback from the earlier episode to try this procedure again, so a new doctor turned up, sat next to me and said "take a deep breath and say aarh . . . Whoosh and out comes the tube on the right . . . not so bad (a dose of morphine before had helped) and yes one more tube inserted into my spine for the drip-feed morphine was also taken out and replaced by a drip on demand with a push-button device, which one could only trigger once every hour, hence leaving me with some highs and lows between shots.

The only other major event left was the removal of all 23 metal clips on my lower chest and stomach areas. One of the nicer nurses was given the task to do the procedure and my little Michelle being only 6½ years of age at that time wanted to stand by me, holding my hand while watching the nurse take out the metal clips one by one. I was very much surprised how Michelle handled all this, even the nurse was amazed, and good old morphine did not fail me.

A few days before my discharge, Dr Geoffrey Ku from Johns Hopkins Cancer Centre came and saw me. He explained that he would be taking on my case for the follow-up Chemo treatment. Johns Hopkins was located at the same hospital within TTSH so we agreed to take up his offer and go along with his recommendations. The treatment however could only start later when I was able to withstand its effects. As I also had to undergo radiation treatment, I would be seeing yet another doctor on this.

Then came the day I was being discharged. After 23 days in the hospital I was set free, along with my bags of medication containing morphine, painkillers, pills for this and pills for that. But who cares I was going home, albeit in a wheelchair as I could only take a few steps at a time (I had slowed down in more ways than one). But the funny thing I could remember is that I still had my big belly, yup still 42 inches even after the operation— but that would all change in time.

We were so touched by the care of all the staff, doctors, nurses and even the cleaner during my stay of 23 days. My little one Michelle made a special drawing to pin up on the notice board, my wife helped me to write a special Thank you card. During one of our many visits back to the hospital, we brought a small picnic basket of kiwifruit, wine & gifts just to show our deepest appreciation. It takes a special type of person to work with terminally ill patients and in my eyes they are all angels.

When we reached home, my mother-in-law had borrowed a wheelchair for me, how thoughtful of her and here she is at age 72 walking around just fine and me at the age of 55 a very tired old man, but still alive and kicking . . . be it only just.

Now if only I could get up those stairs to my bedroom. With the domestic helper Tati, my wife and my little one Michelle pushing me from behind, one managed somehow to make it up. But coming down, I found out later, was 10 times worse.

At least I had new air-conditioning installed at our place, this was again decided by me just before I was admitted into hospital. There were several reasons behind the decision: one, the old air-con leaked and was noisy and not working properly, and two I would have a nice cold room to relax in when I returned home, but the real reason was to ensure it was fixed and gave no trouble to my wife as she would have lots of issues to deal with. If I did not make it and return home, I wanted her not to be troubled over a small issue like the air-con. I knew that if it breaks down or leaks water all over the floor then this small issue would blow up into a big issue and add more stress to her. So I booked in the contractors, arranged for the payment just days before I went into hospital, deal done and all set in motion.

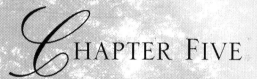

CHAPTER FIVE

The Long Road Ahead—
radiation and chemotheraphy

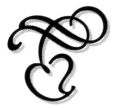

The Long Road Ahead—
radiation and chemotheraphy

I f you have never been to a cancer ward or radiation treatment centre, don't go unless you have too. It is very depressing unless you go to a private clinic like I did for Johns Hopkins where it is all done up like a hotel suite and check-in centre, large armchairs to relax in while you undergo your Chemo treatment via drip feed, Milo and snacks for the family members, etc.; it is somewhat inviting. I did not see many locals there (Southeast Asians) but mainly Middle East patients, and you couldn't tell if they were showing the cancer signs as the women were all covered up in black.

Still the service was good, friendly staff and friendly nurses willing to lend a shoulder to cry on so to speak, they even laughed at some of my jokes (there I go again wearing my magic mask). I think they saw right through me and knew it was my way of coping. Better to laugh than cry right, as *"Grown Men Don't Cry"* . . .

Chemical Warfare

According to my oncologist, Dr Geoffrey Ku, the best time for my Chemo treatment would have been "before" my operation, however the surgeon had a different view and said that my gullet could have closed at any time and choked me to death and/or having Chemo treatment while still having tumours inside of me may make the tumours "swell" thus choking me to death—seems like the surgeon won this medical bout, lucky for me right?

Anyway I was told the best chance of fighting my Cancer would be to use an aggressive form of treatment based on overseas trials in the USA (yet to be published as it was still very much in the early stages) which have shown promising results so far. This treatment would mean that I would come into the clinic for the 2-to-3 hours drip of Chemo cocktail, blood test, etc. once a month, and take home any medication needed as well as these extra strong large pills "custom-made" just for me. Just take 3 in the morning and 3 at night and all would be fine . . . I was led to believe.

On the first day of treatment, all I felt was some discomfort and was a little light-headed, was also tired but other than that it was okay. It must had been due to the morphine I was allowed to take—15 mls every hour for the pain, so I was on a high 24/7. Undergoing this drip feed of cocktails was no sweat. The following morning I had to take my first round of extra strong designer pills. One by one I took them and it was very hard to swallow (not forgetting my insides were turned inside out during the operation just 3 weeks prior) but there I did it. I laid back to rest, and slowly but surely I started to get a reaction. I started to shake and my head started to spin. I started to feel like vomiting so it was time to take the other pills given to me, like anti-vomiting pills and tummy cramp pills and more morphine, but just maybe these pills being as strong as they were, perhaps they just needed more time for my body to accept them?

Then evening came and I had to take these super-duper anti-cancer pills again and yep, the same thing happened. Oh well, maybe after a good night's sleep I should be able to take the pills again, no sweat . . . The next day, as I was being helped downstairs, I could feel myself getting upset with just the thought of taking those pills, yet I forced myself to take them, and yes it came with the same results. So we decided we needed to see the doctor and made an appointment the following day but come evening time, like a true soldier, I forced myself yet again to take the pills. My hands were shaking as I picked up the pill to place into my mouth, a feeling of sickness ran through my body and I had the urge to throw up again, this was all happening before I had taken any one of the pills, let alone three of them. And I had other medication to take. I just could not carry on like this. If this is the so-called best cancer treatment, then I want nothing to do with it. I just hoped and prayed that they had cut out all of the infected cancer tissue and stopped it from spreading.

The very next day I collapsed on the floor and my wife rushed me to the hospital only to find out I was dehydrated due to the pills, and me not eating for the past few days and throwing up what little I had tried to eat. So I was warded yet again in the hospital and had a drip inserted to give me an energy boost which had little effect but at least gave me a fighting chance to semi-recover before the next stage of treatment.

My wife was at a loss of words to support me. I could see it in her eyes how painful this was for her and it seemed unfair that she and my family had to see me go through this. But this was only the beginning and matters took a turn for the worse, much worse.

It was decided these special extra strong Cancer treatment pills were just too much for my body to accept, so Plan B was put into force where I would still be given the monthly special cocktail treatment via drip but I would also be given 24/7 medication also by drip via a tube that had been inserted into my upper left arm previously.

Looking back on the day they inserted this tube, I had been told it was a very simple operation to insert this long tube and it would be done as an outpatient procedure but the trick was that I would be wide awake during the whole procedure looking and watching the surgeon's smallest move. But it turned out to be no biggie, after all I had just come out of a major surgery so a little half-hour operation was nothing, no big deal.

The next stage would be to insert a very large needle into the back of my hand and connect it to a device which held the drip feed bag of the latest cocktail of medication. The device which came in a carry pouch was battery-operated and worked like a timer to inject a dose of medication directly into the tube that was planted into my upper left arm. Now the issue here is the average Asian is small-built and not so tall hence using the same device and tube length to connect from the pouch to my upper arm was just a tad too short.

Well as one sleeps, one normally turns from side to side, in my case I turn a lot and each time I turn I would be woken up with a sharp pain as the tube connected to the pouch was too short and would "tug" at the connection on my arm. I would go to the extent of describing the pain as that of someone trying to yank the tube out of my arm. So to overcome this, I learnt the trick that was when one moved from side to side, one "carries" the pouch with you, and yes you can do this in your sleep, believe it or not. So this would be the "sleep procedure" for the following 3 months. Oh! How wonderful and exciting this would be.

Now the next trick was how to undergo radiation treatment "at the same time as the Chemo treatment". Yes, this was the next phase of my treatment and the hardest.

Microwave Toasting

So arrangements were made for me to see yet another doctor; this time—the radiologist. The department was located in the basement car park of the hospital (just seemed a strange location, but perhaps there's a reason for this, maybe so that any radiation leaks would only affect cars and very few people, if any?). The radiologist was very polite and came across as very caring. He discussed various options and arranged for a MRI, after which I would have another type of scan and get "tattoo" markings on my body (only small blue dots) to pinpoint where the radiation machine would do its job.

Now the issue here was I had the cancer in the mid-chest region and stomach, so I was considered one of the lucky ones where I would get "double" dose of radiation to cover both areas at the same time (but it did not work out that I could get 2 microwave blasts for the price of one). Before any radiation treatment could commence I had to go and get my "cast" fitted, so another appointment was made for this procedure.

When I was informed about the "cast" I did not understand what he was talking about and during our consultation one just either nodded or muttered yes, perhaps not to appear dumb. I expect this was quite normal for most people and only a small number of people would be asking questions.

Here I was again at the Radiation Department, a place where I would hit rock bottom and dread to enter, even with my mask on it was hard to hide my true feelings and to hold back the tears. I would joke and play games on my iPad just so I would not have to look into the eyes of fellow patients in order not to see their deep sadness and pain, and to hide my own. Selfless as it seems, maybe they were also doing the same like me.

So I struggled to stand up to follow a young male nurse who had walked over to me. Both him and my wife helped me to stand with the aid of my trusted walking stick in one hand and my other hand holding my pouch containing the Chemo cocktail being pumped into me every minute. Each day, I began to feel more and more discomfort as the Chemo treatment started to work and take its toll on me. At the same time, it seemed to slow down my recovery from the major operation I had just went through.

We entered a semi-dark room. I somehow laid down on a table where I was put into the most awkward position with both of my arms behind my head, and a nurse holding my Chemo treatment pouch (still connected via a tube to my left upper arm). Then they started to mould this plaster of Paris from the tips of my fingers, down my arm, neck and base of my back, which after 20 minutes or so set rock hard. This was my very own made-to-order cast to be used for each radiation treatment at a special price of only S$1200.

My first radiation treatment, which I refer to as being microwaved or toasted, was scary. I hobbled to the main radiation door, which looked like a type of bank vault door at Fort Knox, the thickness of the door must have been 12-14 inches and the size of the thing looked as though it would take a small army just to open and close it.

At the door, my wife was told she was not allowed to go any further. So I hobbled the last few metres inside and there was my special cast, lying in wait for me, on the raised table. I had to remove my shoes and t-shirt, lie down on my back and somehow fit my arms and fingers into the mould and get "locked" into position, with my tube still connected to my arm and connected to the Chemo pouch. There were 3 staff present, doing all the checks and aligning the radiation points with the recent tattoos on my body. I was told not to move as the radiation machine would rotate around my body. In what I thought was a touching gesture, someone put on some pop music for me. And I wondered . . . why is it so loud? Next minute I was all alone in the room.

Contact

I soon found out how a dinner plate feels like when inside a microwave oven, and the noise of the machine! No wonder the music was so loud. The machine started to rotate and then it stopped at a pre-set position on my chest—zap, zap, zap . . . then it moved to the next position—zap, zap, zap . . . then the next and the next until it completed the whole cycle all in all about 20 minutes.

I felt a little bit warm inside of me but other than that I was okay. I remember thinking is this it? Piece of cake, I could handle this AND my Chemo treatment at the same time, nothing to worry about.

I was helped off the table, helped to get dressed and helped to the waiting area outside where my loved one waited for me. I could see she was eager to hear how it was. I just smiled and said it's a piece of cake no problem, so after booking our next session (I had a total of 42 radiation treatments) we walked back to the car.

It was not long after reaching home I started to feel "strange". Somehow I had gotten semi-accustomed to the side effects of the Chemo, and the pains from the surgery incisions on my stomach and back, but this feeling of being "toasted" and a warm glow inside of me was not a pleasant feeling.

My radiation treatment was 5 days a week with a break over the weekends for recovery. This went on for approximately six weeks. Each time I turned up for treatment I would cry inside. I tried my best to ensure I wore my mask to hide my true feelings from others. I would try to play my war game on my iPad, just to distract myself from what was about to happen.

During radiation, the parts of your body being zapped will cause your skin to be "roasted", much like a sunburn. At the same time, the chemotherapy will compromise your immune system, making you more subject to getting viruses like catching a cold or flu, hence even Fr John Sim, my church priest, advised me "not" to come to church for Mass as I would most likely fall ill and complications may set in.

Certain radiation sessions would last up to 40 minutes, with small 5-minute breaks and recalibration taking place. But these were far and few in between as the normal session would last about 20 minutes at a time. I tried my best to listen to the music played at full blast in order to drown out the eerie noise of the radiation machine, so the patient doesn't freak out! But it really did not help much. Then I started to count the cycles of the machine as it zapped away at me like a ray-gun. That just made me more scared, so I started to say the Lord's Prayer and somehow I kept forgetting the words and had to start all over again and again, but in no time at all the 20 minutes flew by, and the session seemed to be over in like 5 minutes. So from that day onwards, I would say the Lord's Prayer every time I underwent the treatment. I regarded it as a way that the good Lord had wanted me to communicate with him and to receive his power of healing.

"I waited patiently for the Lord; He turned to me and heard my cry.
He lifted me out of the slimy pit, Out of the mud and mire;
He set my feet on a rock and gave me a firm place to stand.
He put a new song in my mouth, A hymn of praise to our God.
Many will see and fear and put their trust in the Lord."
—Psalm 40:1-3

I had to rest all the time and conserve my energy. I was unable to eat any food for 3 months other than oranges and ice-cream 3-4 times a day, hence this was the main reason why I lost 30kg in 3 months! I would not recommend this way of dieting to anyone. I would wake up 2-3 times a night vomiting and shaking, feeling hot and cold. The effects of the radiation and Chemo treatment were so harsh that I would hide myself in the toilet and cry just to let out my sorrows so that my family would not see me in such a poor state of mind and body.

A few times I would sit at the table, look at the food and start to fight back the tears. My face would turn red and my little Michelle would just hold my hand or stroke my arm to give me comfort. I would excuse myself to lie down without touching any of the food. I just could not look at the food, let alone eat it.

There was one time just before my treatment, I told the radiology staff that I had chest pains and asked if I could take my morphine medication (we have our own stack of medication prescribed by the surgeon including morphine that my wife carries around with her just in case of emergencies). Could he go outside and get it from my wife? I saw his face turn almost white. He told me to sit down and he went outside only to appear again with two doctors who began to examine me and start asking a whole lot of questions. I think they suspected I was having a heart attack! I found out later that this had happened to one of their patients before. I assured them that all I had was a bad and sleepless night, and been having the same type of pains on and off for quite a while and my heart was strong (well that is what the doctors and nurses said after a number of ECGs and scans in the ward previously). But they wanted me to go up to the A&E for a check-up. I said no, I just wanted to get this microwave treatment over and done with for the day. In the end I had to sign a waiver that I would not hold the hospital accountable if I should pass away on the radiation table. They put a monitor around my ankle while I was undergoing the radiation treatment, and yes I did manage to take a swig of my morphine to help with the pain. I would sometimes shock people as I would just take a swig from the bottle for liquid medications; no need to pour into a plastic holder, waste of time.

As I underwent the radiation and chemo treatment, I was getting weaker and weaker. I needed the use of the wheelchair and people to help me in almost all my daily activities. Our helper Tati also had to give me a massage once every few days.

I recall there was a time I was almost warded again. It happened close to midnight and I was in so much pain despite the double dose of morphine and tummy cramp pills. They just did not work. In the end I was rushed to the hospital's A&E.

After being examined by a quiet young female doctor I was told I needed an urgent operation as my intestines were blocked and could burst at any time. She wanted to put a tube down me but I refused (I just had enough of tubes being inserted into my body by this time) and she raised her voice and said "I am trying to save your life. Listen to me!" But I still refused to have any tube put inside of me while I was awake.

I was wheeled to the observation area and told to rest while waiting for the doctors from the Operating Theatre to examine me. The staff were ready to wheel me straight into the Operating Theatre if needed.

Out came a group of three doctors all dressed in their gowns and masks, looking at me, prodding me and asking a few questions before they went away to discuss what to do. I was left not only in pain, light-headed and a bit on cloud nine (having taken double swigs of morphine). I wondered what the hell was happening, am I going under the knife again or what? Then I was moved to another area and someone else took my place (a bit like a conveyer belt all lined up for the knife action to begin inside the magic room) but as time went by I started to feel a bit better and by 5am in the morning I was ok to leave the A&E and go back home.

So I was trapped into a routine. Weekdays I get my double dose of microwave zapping, chemotherapy was a 24/7 dose, and every three weeks I get to sit in an armchair and have a new cocktail given via a drip during a 1 to 2 hour session with the most painful part being the changing of the dressing on my upper arm. Each time they took off the dressing, they would also take off a layer of my skin, not forgetting that both during the day and night, I would be vomiting every few hours, taking morphine and other countless pills.

"God wants me to Suffer; I think he's preparing
me for something important
Something that I will come to understand in his time
It is a privilege to cry, it means
I'm among his special Children"

~ As Grown Men Don't Cry ~

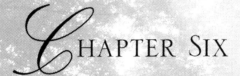 CHAPTER SIX

Angels sent to Watch over me

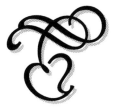

Angels sent to Watch over me

I remember Fr John Sim, our local Priest from Church of the Risen Christ, who came to see me in late December to give me another anointing and blessing. He would arrange for someone to visit me weekly to give me Holy Communion.

> *(Holy Communion refers to the <u>Eucharist</u> and the wine that some Christians take as a symbol of the body and blood of Christ, during a portion of a church service. In Roman <u>Catholicism</u>, Holy Communion is not simply symbolic of the body of Christ, but it is as well the body of Christ. It is a sacrament. Sacrament in Catholicism is described as the symbol of the thing and the thing itself. This means when practicing Catholics take Holy Communion; it has been transformed through prayer into the physical body of Christ. They are*

*thus taking Christ within themselves. Source http://
www.wisegeek.com/what-is-holy-communion.htm)*

The following week I received a phonecall from a person named Robert, a Communion Minister from the Church. Extraordinary Ministers of Holy Communion to the Sick and Homebound (also known as Ministers of Care) have a role in sharing the Church's total ministry to the sick after the manner of Jesus. In bringing Communion to the sick and homebound, the Minister of Care represents Christ and manifests faith and charity on behalf of the whole community toward those who cannot be present at Sunday Mass.

This is the first time I have ever been visited by anyone at home from the Church (other than the Priest who just came a week before) and again I did not know what to expect. The timing was set for a Wednesday 10 am, so it would give me time to recover slightly from my morning sickness, have a wash and tidy myself up, get helped downstairs and be resting on the settee and waiting.

Right on time this Robert turned up. As I was not strong enough to get up from the settee, our domestic helper Tati let him in. Within a few minutes I felt at ease and found this person to be very caring, kind and considerate. He was not worried at all that I could not sit up, read the Bible passage or remember any of the Mass, he took all this in his stride, thanked me and gave me a blessing and told me to just rest as he could see his own way out. I felt so calm and at peace, and my pains just seemed to be just more bearable.

I looked forward to these weekly meetings and to receive Holy Communion and over the weeks I grew stronger until one such day I was able to meet Robert at the door and let him in.

He was so surprised and happy for me as I now had the strength to get up and walk to the door all by myself. What progress! Praise be to God! And I found myself also thanking God more and more, but one thing I never forgot to say was to thank God for sending me an Angel to look after me in my time of need.

I got so encouraged that I would start to recover from this cancer I even arranged for a contractor to do the extension to our balcony and to remodel my son's bedroom, just a little project to keep me busy and to take the focus away from the radiation and chemo treatment along with all the side effects. I was often too tired and weak to bother about the noise and dust but having this little (actually, not so little) project to focus on took away the worry and some of the pain. During this period, I remember always wanting to sip water due to my dry mouth. I could hardly drink any decent amount; I could only sip and wet my lips, it was all I needed every hour almost day and night.

There came a time when my hair started to fall out, I cried for hours and felt ashamed, *Grown men don't cry* . . . or at least not in front of my own family, as I had to be strong for them. I decided to buy an electric handheld mattress cleaner so that each morning our domestic helper Tati would clean up all the hair and leave no evidence. I also decided and managed to somehow hobble down to the local barber and get my head almost shaved bald. My daughter Sharon brought me a gentlemen's cap so I would not be so embarrassed out in public.

As the weeks went by and during my ups and downs, (mood swings and depression being one of the uncontrollable side effects of Cancer treatment—hence having to take anti-depression medication) and throughout the renovations with all the dust, dirt, contractors coming in and out, and our place being in a complete mess, Robert never failed to turn up. He never said anything negative and took all this upheaval in his stride—here was a person whom he never knew before, who having just gotten over a major operation, and fighting to survive radiation and chemo treatment, was now at the same time somehow taking on a renovation project inside his own home which he could hardly walk around in. He must have thought the pills had affected my brain and left me with no sense whatever.

"But that what's makes an Angel special"

So two months into my radiation and chemo, I had the strength to venture outside my home on very short trips of up to 1 to 2 hours at a time. As long as my wife had armed herself with all my medication, we would feel semi-safe to step outside the door and go somewhere other than to the hospital.

It would be a strange feeling whenever I meet someone, be it my wife's friends, my friends or even some of the family, once you were labelled with the Big C somehow people don't know what to say to you; they would try to avoid you or not look you directly in the eye. I often wondered why. Maybe they thought it was like getting Hand, Foot & Mouth Disease (HFMD) or most likely they did't know what to say. But it is still me, just got this slight issue (well maybe not so slight after all).

To me I was okay talking about my Cancer but I would not be the one to bring up the subject. If someone was willing to ask me "How are you doing?", I would just say "okay". If they asked about the treatment, then I say a bit more and end with the fact that I am coping with it. But very few people I came into contact with asked about my Cancer. It seemed to be the unwritten rule not to talk about the Big C, it's a no-no.

With this reaction I decided that when the time was right for me to get back to work, be it part-time or full-time (I was in real estate a few years before I found out I had cancer), I would keep the illness to myself as I did not want the "pity" card to be played and wanted to undertake any work based on my own abilities at the time, however restricted it may be.

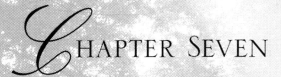

CHAPTER SEVEN

The Second Wave—
A test of faith

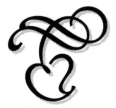

The Second Wave—A test of faith

What was not so unusual were the expected side effects as I had been forewarned; be it due to the major operation, the radiation, chemo, the monthly blood tests, etc. I even expected to have ALL the known common and maybe some of the not so common side effects, more so as I was one of the lucky ones to have both radiation and chemo at the same time, both in high dosages.

What I didn't expect was losing my step now and then, blacking out (I expected being dizzy or light-headed, but not black-outs), and having a very sharp pain in the mid-section to the right. I brought this up with my gastrologist not once but twice and after examining me, he would come to the conclusion I was still recovering from my major operation and it may be the pain from my ribs being cut (found out they cut two of my ribs to get access to my insides), so I would just get more medication and make yet another appointment in a month's time.

This worried me and the dizziness and pain only seemed to be getting worse over time. So at my next appointment with my oncologist I brought up the same issues and he agreed to make an appointment to get a MRI brain scan and spine scan the following week. And when the time came for the two scans I just cracked a few jokes like "I wonder if they find any grey matter inside my head?" or "Knock knock! Anyone or anything inside?" This was of course to give myself assurance and not to worry my wife, but deep inside I was really worried, what if they find something? What if the cancer had spread to my nervous system? What if . . .

So as I lay down for yet another one of the scans (never gets any easier), I was given ear plugs and a face strap (to isolate my head) and had to hold my arms behind my head (at the same time hold onto my chemo pouch still connected to the tube in my arm) then in I went.

Now just imagine standing next to a jack hammer while it is breaking up the road or concrete. Now imagine this happening inside a tunnel . . . you get the picture? But you can't move, you can't talk, your ears are ringing and yes, I am praying.

After the one run (scan number one), out I came and got re-positioned and then put through the whole process again . . . nice one. But the good thing was it was over within 30 minutes and I walked out and met my wife waiting for me. "How was it?" she asked. "Piece of cake," I answered and quickly looked away.

The results came back and they found grey matter inside, yes I have some brains in my head. But no problems were found and nothing to worry about, so what was causing these side effects that no one could answer? So apart from seeing the surgeon, the radiation and the Cancer doctors, I was told to see the Pain

Management doctor for consultation, so they think I am now going crazy, is it? But ok I play along and see yet another doctor. What did I have to lose?

A few days before the appointment I received a rather long "questionnaire" booklet on my own pain assessment, somehow it reminded me of the trick questions you get at some job interviews or a IQ test, but I completed it and took it along for the appointment with this Doctor Who.

Well it turned out this doctor after seeing me for only 15 minutes and doing some prodding with a needle, feather, pen, etc. to test my reaction to feeling sharp and not-so-sharp objects knew exactly what was wrong. It appears during my 5-hour major operation that was done some six months back, that while they were cutting away sections of my ribs they also cut some nerves leaving the nerve ends raw, hence the continuous pain. Not what the gastrorologist was saying, that the pain was due to the healing process of my remaining stomach.

This problem I was told could be easily corrected during a day surgery but may only result in reducing the pain by up to 70% and may only last 2 to 3 years. I quickly said let's go for it, anything is better than what I was experiencing then. So yet another appointment was made for this day surgery. I really did not know what to expect but how much worse could it be after all I had gone through so far?

Then came the day I had to go in for the procedure. I woke up early and prayed that God would guide the doctor's hands to heal me. On arrival I was promptly asked to change into the pre-op gown and as I lay there waiting on the hospital bed, flashbacks to the previous operation were fast and furious but I kept praying and asking for strength.

Inside the operation theatre, I was told to lay face down, head on a pillow, and arms to my side. As explained by the doctor, I was to be awake the entire time during the procedure. How nice and exciting this was going to be! I needed to tell the doctor the intensity of the pain I was feeling, ranging from a low of 1 to a high of 10. After numbing the area of my spine, a rod would be inserted and a wire connected to it. An electric current will pass through to the nerve to locate the damaged one. This would be repeated 4 to 5 times in order to isolate which nerve needed to be "corrected".

So the fun began. While both my arms were held down by two nurses, the procedure went from one nerve to the other, which had me shouting out "three", "four", etc. until the real awakening happened and I screamed "10" and again "10". I felt like screaming 50 or 100 at that point. "Yes! That's good! I found the damaged nerves." I heard the doctor say. "Now relax while we run the electric current for 20 minutes and do the same for the next nerve." Now how is one to relax knowing you are being "fried" and "electrocuted" at the same time!

So I lay there saying the Lord's Prayer and after the 20 minutes were up, the second procedure was completed. I was cleaned up and sent out to the recovery area where my wife was waiting to see me. A few minutes later the doctor came to see me and asked "How are you doing?" and I just replied "okay". But he then asked me to sit up and he tested the affected area for signs of pain and to my amazement, the pain had almost disappeared. "Job well done!" I said and "Praise be to God!".

I know this was a test of my faith and seeing that I still believed in him, God was merciful and had rewarded me. God only gives us enough pain knowing what we can endure and overcome. At times it may seem to be overwhelming but it is a reminder of how much he suffered and died on the Cross for us.

> *"The Lord is good to those whose hope is in him,*
> *To the one who seeks him."*
> —Lamentations 3:25

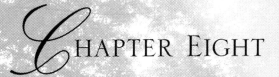

CHAPTER EIGHT

The Four Doctor Who(s)—
Miracle Workers

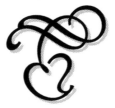

The Four Doctor Who(s)—
Miracle Workers

During the past 12 months I had to undergo a lot of changes in my life, with a lot of pain and despair. I searched for hope. Not only in medical terms, physically or mentally, but also in faith and believing there's a purpose in all this and it is all according to God's Plan for us.

As any committed Christian would know, in times like this, all we needed to do was to utter Jesus' name and every evil spirit will flee. For me I tried to call out the name of Jesus but seemed to be struggling until finally I managed to call out to Jesus during my darkest times. The first time was during the radiation treatment while undergoing chemo. He answered me and allowed me to have the strength to endure the ordeal and come to him.

I must admit that I was not such a good Christian nor a strong believer. I would go along with my wife and mother-in-law to Church and attend some Church events, but it was not until I was tested and allowed to cry, yes *Grown Men Can Cry*, that I was allowed to experience the Lord's blessings.

After my 23 days in hospital, my recovery period at home lasted three weeks before I started my chemotherapy and radiation treatments. With both treatments happening together, I would have doctor consultations weekly at first and then it was extended to every month, then every 3 months, then every six months. Seeing four different specialists on such a regular basis, I got to know the hospital inside and out, and had a growing respect for the doctors and nurses for what they do.

Doctor One—Gastrointestinal Surgeon

My surgeon is one of the most well-respected in his field. I was told many times how lucky I was to have this doctor to look after me. This doctor would prescribe my reflux, tummy pains, anti-sickness, and extra strong painkiller medication.

Doctor Two—Medical Oncologist

Medical oncologists are one of the most common types of oncologists. They specialise in the treatment of solid tumours, usually with chemotherapy or via referral to a surgeon for removal of the tumour.

This is the doctor whom I really got close to. He was the one who prescribed my chemotherapy treatment and was always willing to hear my on-going complaints. He tried his best to not only give me medical support but was a listening ear. As operation costs and on-going medical treatment was touching the S$100,000 mark and climbing, and due to financial issues, I had to apply for a downgrading from private patient to subsidised patient (a very degrading process with the welfare department).

This doctor called me and he was still willing to oversee my on-going chemotherapy treatment at Tan Tock Seng Hospital.

At one point I was having a very hard time with the insurance company for my hospitalisation claim, he openly offered to write a letter to the insurance company to help process my claims as soon as possible. He actually wrote two letters and the insurance company agreed to pay out 75% of my bills (be it almost one year later).

So when he left to return to New York, USA, after almost 18 months of treatment, I was very sad as of all the doctors who have helped me, this doctor was very outstanding and had saved my life, so I just had to write to him to give him my thanks and God's blessing on him.

This doctor again would always make sure I had sufficient medication prescribed by the other doctors as well as ample liquid morphine, mouth wash and cream to fight the effects of the chemotherapy treatment.

Doctor Three—Radiation Oncologist

A radiation oncologist is similar to a medical oncologist, but specialises in treating cancers with radiation.

This doctor was also very professional and understanding. The side effects of radiation can be very extreme but the caring nature shown had helped me during this very difficult time. This doctor would re-confirm I had sufficient pills as well as cream/lotion for my skin affected by the radiation.

Doctor Four—Pain management doctor

This doctor would prescribe me my nerve pain medication. Surgery is often considered the court of last resort for pain: when all else fails, cut the nerve endings. Surgery can bring about instant, almost magical release from pain. But surgery may also destroy other sensations as well, or, inadvertently, become the source of new pain. Further, relief is not necessarily permanent. After 6 months or a year, pain may return.

(Source: http://seniorhealth.about.com/library/conditions/ blchronicpain7.htm)

This is the doctor who undertook the correction of my damaged nerves to reduce my on-going chronic pain which is totally different from what I would say normal pain feels like, like recovery from the operation, broken bones, tooth removal, etc.

Chronic pain is different. Chronic pain persists. Fiendishly, uselessly, pain signals keep firing in the nervous system for weeks, months, even years. There may have been an initial mishap—a sprained back, a serious infection from which you've long since recovered. There may be an on-going cause of pain-arthritis, cancer, ear infection. But some people suffer chronic pain in the absence of any past injury or evidence of body damage. Whatever the cause, chronic pain is real, unremitting, and demoralizing.

(Source: http://seniorhealth.about.com/library/conditions/ blchronicpain1.htm)

So all in all I have Four Doctor Who(s) to see, countless medication—I am down to 12 pills per day, nerve pills, plus some extra vitamins, and a supply of pain and tummy cramp pills when I need them—as well as numerous CT scans and/or MRI scans, let alone endless blood tests, etc. (why do they need five tubes of blood every time?) But that said I am most grateful that the good Lord had guided them during their treatment of me.

I must also mention the countless nurses who have helped me, especially the group of nurses in the Cancer ward, where after my Chemo treatment was finished, we surprised them all by giving them a small box of kiwifruits from this Kiwi guy whom they had helped.

"Jesus said unto her,
I am the resurrection, and the life:
He that believeth in me, though he were dead, yet shall he live."
—John 11:25

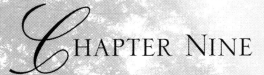

CHAPTER NINE

The Journey Continues—
Life carries on

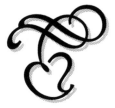

The Journey Continues—
Life carries on

After each fall we must pick ourselves up and carry on, no matter what. Remember when you were a young child and maybe one of your parents would be teaching you how to ride a bicycle and you fall over? You would be told to get back onto the bike and overcome your fears; no matter how many times you fall, you must get back on and master it.

As you grow older, you are faced with many challenges in life, some more extreme than others. Like everything in life, willpower is a learned skill, a mental muscle that people need to exercise.

The quickest way I learnt willpower was to force myself to actually do something and not to feel sorry for myself or have others feel pity for me. I was told I could only plan ahead for the next three months during the early stages of my Cancer treatment as the chances of me surviving beyond that time period was low. Yet I decided to arrange certain small projects to do in our house, like replacement of all our air-conditioning units just days before I went into hospital for my major operation. And after returning home to recover and during my chemo and radiation treatment, I was focused on renovations in our living room to extend our balcony and to re-model my son's bedroom.

I refused to accept a three month window of life, even when this was later extended to six months. I was planning what to do for the next one year and beyond. This is not to say I did not have times when I was struggling with sadness and depression but my deepening understanding of spiritual matters helped me a great deal, and I am still learning until this day.

Return to Work

I was thankful that an old friend Colin who knew my on-going battles with Cancer and my plans to get back to some sort of normal life offered me a position in a newly setup division in a Retail Real Estate company where he would be a Division Director and asked that I follow him. Of course I explained I am half the man I used to be (half the size and half the strength) and will find it hard-going and will restrict my performance. However he stood firm and assured me that he would look after me and in no time I would be back to my normal self.

It was quite timely, as they say when one door closes another one opens. So I joined and convinced 5 to 6 other people to join with me to give him support, but on one condition: my illness and the Big C word was never to be told to others. I wanted to be able to stand on my own two feet and did not want favours due to my having Cancer.

Well, it turned out okay. Each day I would be wearing my mask to hide my emotional feelings, more so when I was experiencing pain and having to hide to take my medications every few hours. It got to a stage where I was so exhausted I would ask my wife to drive me to the showroom and pick me up. Even during my bouts of depression I continued to hide my feelings and my pains and carry on like nothing was wrong. But at times I could see myself falling into a trap, getting stressed about a situation not of my doing and letting rip (blowing my top, losing my cool, bursting out in anger, etc.). It took me days of praying to realise certain things are to be and are outside of your control, no need to be worried and angry about some bad apple who is going against the system and being dishonest, that Senior Management tended to look the other way, as in the end all of us would be judged and had to answer for our sins.

Live our lives the best we can, help others when we can and believe in the good, as good always wins over evil. When I realised this, I felt a great sense of relief like a big burden was lifted from my shoulders and by writing this book I feel more at ease with who I am, what I am, what I can do and not do, and the world around me.

Dreams

I too have dreams. I dream that I wake up one morning without any pains, and have breakfast without feeling sick afterwards. I dream I would be able to go through a whole day without thinking of my limitations due to my illness. I dream of being able to do a full day's work without the need of hiding in a corner to take my medication. But most of all I dream of seeing my children grow up and get married, and start their own family and hold my grandchildren in my arms, be able to talk to them, play with them and teach them the many lessons of life and to never stop dreaming.

Many years back I met my good friend Bill who had joined me in RCIA at the Church of the Risen Christ. We had planned to do some business together in the Philippines as well as in Indonesia and other undeveloped countries with the aim to help the very poor, in projects like building basic infrastructures, schools, hospitals, low cost homes, etc. This was not to be on a grand scale but where it would have the most impact. Until this day Bill is still in the Philippines trying to find ways to make this happen. We pray to God that he will show us the way and allow us to fulfil our dreams to help others.

I also dream that technology will continue to advance in discovering ways to treat and cure all types of Cancer, for both young and old, men and woman, so people all over the world do not have to go through and endure the pain and heart-breaking treatment(s) that I and others had to.

> *"I know the plans I have for you, declares the Lord,*
> *Plans to prosper you and not to harm you,*
> *Plans to give you hope and a future."*
> —Jeremiah 29:11

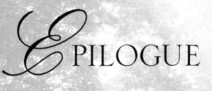

EPILOGUE

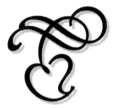

No matter how hard we fall, how deep into despair we go and how much pain we endure, we must always have hope.

If you trust in the Lord, then you will know he only gives as much pain as he knows we can bear; that he has a plan for every one of us and in his time he will allow us to experience his great joyfulness. Having a relationship with Jesus allows us to have a good spiritual footing and to fall back to the basics of who we are and where we should be as we struggle with all the issues. It is never too late to start; sometimes we have to endure great pains and hardships and learn many lessons along the way, but in the end we achieve peace in the understanding of his passion.

Overcoming Cancer is a fight of the body, mind and spirit. While doctors can take care of our medical aspects, it is up to each one of us as individuals to have hope and willpower. Be it a good friend or your spouse as your pillar of support (in my case

I had both, my wife was my pillar keeping me upright and my friend Roy was always positive giving me advice and support, even during his own struggles of ill health and work), or your doctor or your priest, there will be someone there for you as long as you are open to receiving help.

At the time of writing this book, it has been 20 months since my major operation, radiation and chemotherapy treatment. I am nearing the magic 2-year mark where one has been told that beyond this milestone, chances of survival greatly increases up to 70% to reach the next big milestone of five years. After the 5th year you are considered in "remission" but not cured of Cancer. Doctors almost never use the term cure; rather, they usually talk about remission.

Complete remission means that there are no symptoms and no signs that can be identified to indicate the presence of cancer. However, even when a person is in remission, there may be microscopic collections of cancer cells that cannot be identified by current techniques. This means that even if a person is in remission, they may, at some future time, experience a recurrence of their cancer.[2]

So life goes on, we all have our own share of burdens to carry and must accept that's how we are, but how we live depends on each individual and whether they follow the path that is set out for us. And remember *Grown Men Can Cry* and life carries on even after having Cancer.

"*Weeping may endure for a night, but joy cometh in the morning.*"
—Psalms 30:5

---

[2]   http://www.everydayhealth.com/blog/zimney-health-and-medical-news-you-can-use/cancer-cure-vs-remission/

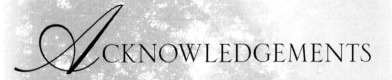

ACKNOWLEDGEMENTS

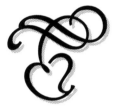

Throughout my long journey I have met many warm-hearted people, strangers who have become friends, professionals like doctors and nurses who have cared for me with kindness and love that is beyond what is expected, and many priests and Church members who have prayed for me and over me endlessly. I can only list a few here, but my heart and love goes out to all.

First and foremost I give thanks to my Lord who allowed me to accept his grace and blessings. My deepest thanks and love to my wife Karen who has been a pillar and rock of support and understanding during my highest joys and lowest moments; she has kept faith in me during the darkest times. My thanks also to my family—my sons Chris and Shane, my daughters Sharon and Michelle, who came and supported me during my 25 days in hospital, I love them all as they are the reason why I fought this Cancer tooth and nail, and not forgetting my mother-in-law "Cecilia Fong" who though in her 70s, went selflessly from church to church attending masses for the sick, prayer groups for the sick and arranging for many groups to pray over me.

For the staff at Tan Tock Seng Hospital in Singapore who have acted with professionalism and kindness, to many in the parishes of Church of the Risen Christ (Toa Payoh) and Church of Saint Michael (Serangoon) who prayed for me, especially Fr. John Sim, Fr. Kamil Kamus and Fr. Angel who were very dear to me and very understanding. They anointed me, and asked our Lord to help and protect me during my Operation and treatment.

Special thanks goes to Jeanette who heads the Ministry F.R.E.E (Faith, Renewal, Exploration & Evangelisation) at the Church of the Risen Christ, a faith formation ministry which both Karen and I belong to since it was founded in 2007. The whole group has kept me in their prayers. We continue to join the video teachings and sessions about the Word of the Lord.

I must not forget one of the special Angels sent by the Lord—Robert from Church of the Risen Christ, who had come to visit me in the hospital ward and to my home to give me Holy Communion every week without fail until I was well enough to go to church in the wheelchair and attend Mass.

The whole experience has led me to do some soul searching and to be able to "hear" the word of the Lord and experience his suffering. Not long after my recovery when I started to do some part-time Real Estate work, I met a guy Robin who introduced me to a product called TH17, an Anti-Cancer Natural Health Supplement slated to be launched in Singapore in late 2013. I began taking the Mangosteen juice together with Th17 supplements, and to my surprise, I had, within 3 months, started to gain some weight and was feeling a lot more energetic. This has inspired me to start and support a Charity and to help other Cancer sufferers to try this new health supplement. I have recently restarted my own business and have included this product into my website www.globalfocusbiz.com to help others find out more about this exciting new and approved product. You can email th17.care@gmail.com or visit us on Facebook under TH17 Natural Care Products.

For those who prayed for me, and who have helped me in one way or another (I know there are many of you out there whom I have not mentioned by name) I say God Bless You all and thanks from the bottom of my heart for your gift of love.

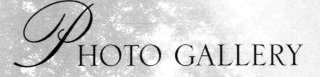

PHOTO GALLERY

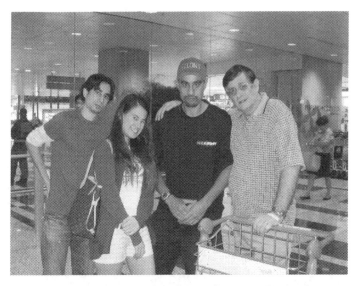

November 2010—Chris flew in from New Zealand to give me support. Here we are welcoming Chris at the airport. (L-R): Shane, Sharon and Chris.

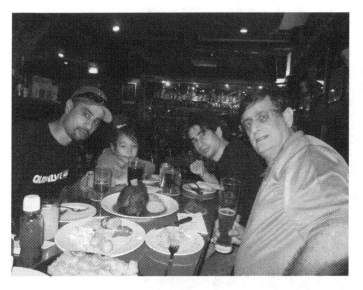

A night out with the family at our neighbourhood German pub. (L-R): Chris, Michelle and Shane.

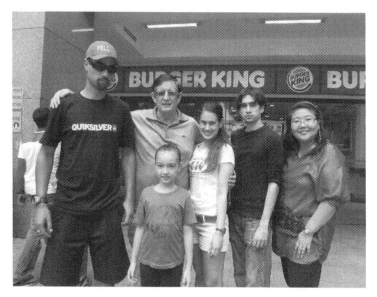

A family photo before the operation (L-R):
Chris, Michelle, Sharon, Shane and Karen.

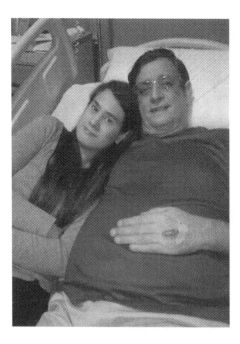

Sharon snuggles up to me
at the hospital, the night
before the operation.

After the operation, more tubes and needles in me than I thought possible.

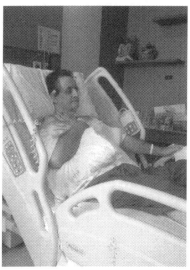

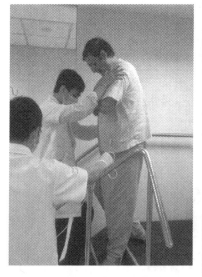

Who would have thought walking down the stairs could be terrifying!

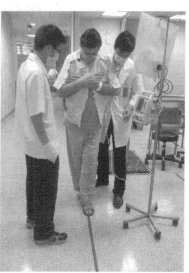

A very patient and caring physiotherapist who really let me do things one step at a time.

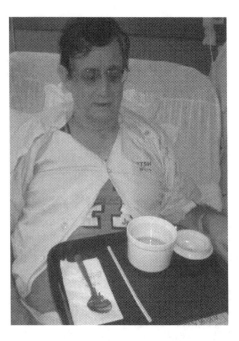

Is that all they are
going to feed me?

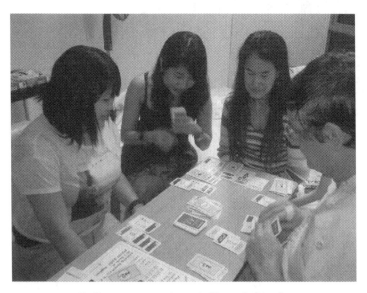

Feeling young again with Sharon's friends,
I am touched that they came to keep an old man
company. (L-R): Grace, Valerie and Sharon.

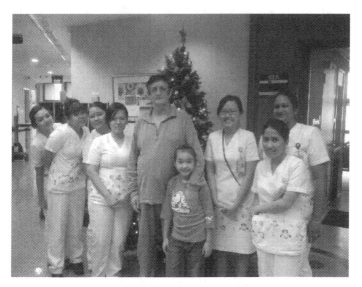

The amazing nursing staff at Tan Tock Seng
Hospital. Their ability to weather my moods
was simply amazing. Thank you nurses.

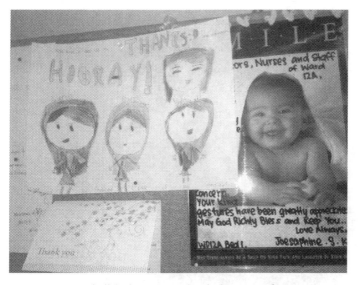

Michelle's drawing to thank the nurses for
taking such good care of Daddy.

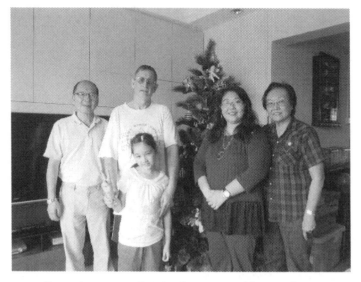

December 2010—Fr John Sim came to bless our home during Christmas. Fr John's anointing and prayers was a comfort before and after my operation. (L-R): Fr John Sim, Michelle, Karen and mother-in-law, Cecilia.

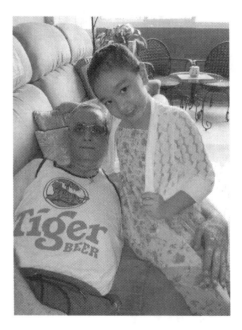

December 2010—The first round of chemotherapy had turned my hair white.

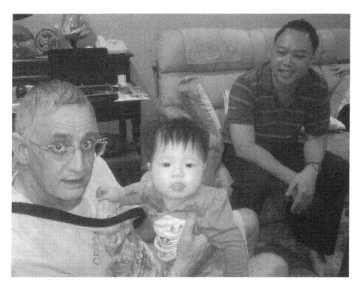

Me and my chemo pouch which I had to wear all day and night.
Church friends Jeffrey and Amelia came to visit with baby Estee.

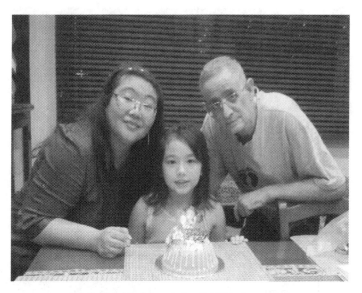

Michelle's birthday, 9 April 2011. I survived
the Chemotherapy and Radiation.

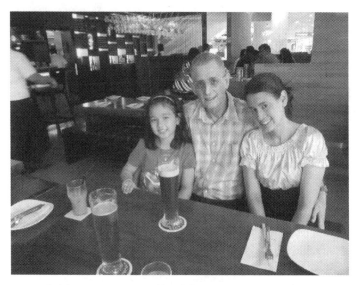

Celebrating 2011 April birthdays at Vivocity: Michelle (9 April), Mine (14 April) and Sharon (29 April).

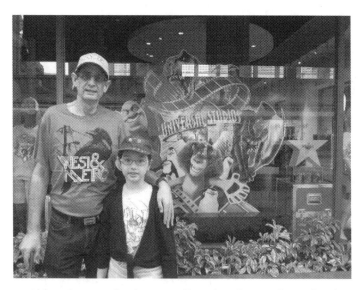

Although energy levels were still at a low, I spent the weekend with Karen and Michelle at Resorts World Sentosa and visited Universal Studios Singapore—June 2011.

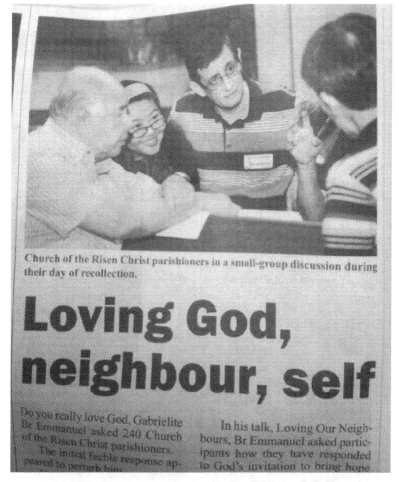

Church of the Risen Christ parishioners in a small-group discussion during their day of recollection.

Loving God, neighbour, self

Do you really love God, Gabrielite Br Emmanuel asked 240 Church of the Risen Christ parishioners.

The initial feeble response appeared to perturb him.

In his talk, Loving Our Neighbours, Br Emmanuel asked participants how they have responded to God's invitation to bring hope

A joy to be participating in church activities again. A moment captured by the local Catholic newspaper; little did they know my journey was indeed about Loving God, neighbour and self.

Featured with permission from Catholic News Singapore, Issue 23 September 2012.

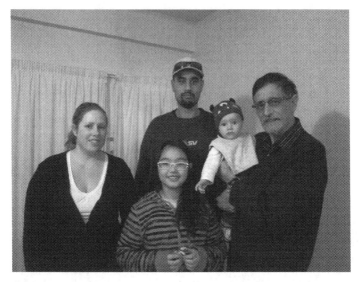

A long-awaited trip to New Zealand to see Chris and his wife Emma, and the first grandson of the family, Connor—June 2013.

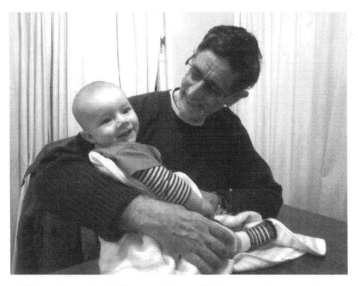

What a joy to hold Connor Ashton Roberts, my first grandson, born on 31 December 2012. One of my wishes have come through.

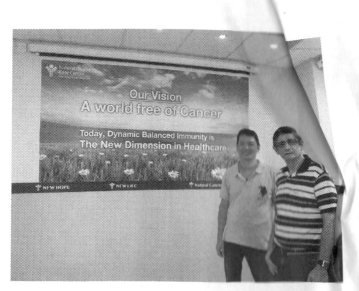

Envisioning a world free of Cancer with Simon,
owner of the Natural Cancer Care Center (Singapore)—2013

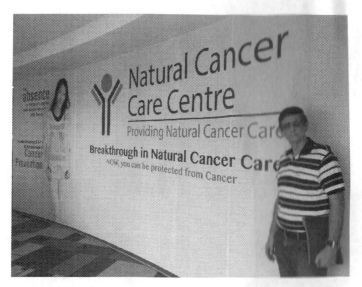

Outside the Natural Cancer Care Centre (Singapore)—2013